Initiation into Egyptian Yoga and Neterian Spirituality Workbook for Beginning and Advancing Aspirants

based on the Book

INITIATION INTO EGYPTIAN YOGA AND NETERIAN SPIRITUALITY

by Sebai Dr. Muata Ashby

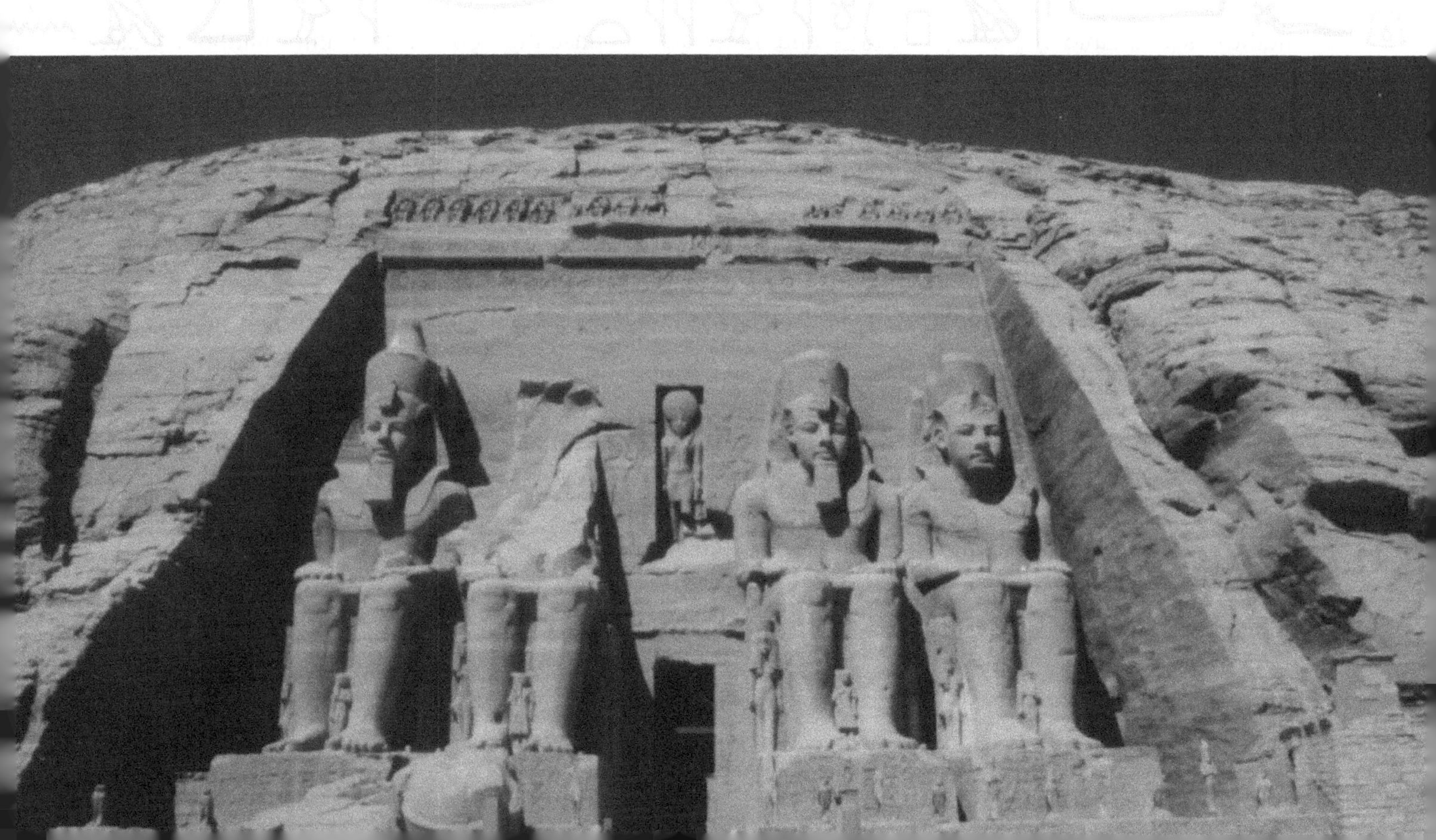

Initiation into Egyptian Yoga and Neterian Spirituality Workbook for Beginning and Advancing Aspirants

based on the Book

INITIATION INTO EGYPTIAN YOGA AND NETERIAN SPIRITUALITY

by Sebai Dr. Muata Ashby

Cruzian Mystic Books
Sema Yoga
P.O.Box 570459
Miami, Florida, 33257
(305) 378-6253 Fax: (305) 378-6253

First U.S. edition 2014-2016

All rights reserved. No part of this book may be used or reproduced in any manner whatsoever without written permission (address above) except in the case of brief quotations embodied in critical articles and reviews. All inquiries may be addressed to the address above.

The author is available for group lectures and individual counseling. For further information contact the publisher.

Ashby, Muata
Initiation Into Egyptian Yoga and Neterian Spirituality Workbook For Beginning and Advancing Aspirants.
ISBN: 1-884564-85-2

Library of Congress Cataloging in Publication Data

1 Yoga Philosophy, 2 Egyptian Philosophy 3 African Mythology 4 Meditation, 5 Self Help.

Table of Contents

- THE SEMA INSTITUTE AND 5
- TEMPLE OF SHETAUT NETER 5
  - Sema Institute of Yoga 5
  - AUTHOR Sebai Muata Ashby Ph. D., D.D., P.C., Y.U. 6
  - Hemit Dja Un Nefert Ashby 7
- A Brief History of Shetaut Neter 8
  - Early Beginnings: The First Religion 8
  - The Term Kamit and the Origins of the Ancient Egyptians 10
    - The Hieroglyphic Text for the Name Qamit 10
- Who Were the Ancient Egyptians and What is Yoga Philosophy? 12
- What is Initiation? 16
  - The Initiatic Way of Education 16
    - PERSONAL ASSESSMENT 22
- Yoga in Ancient Egypt 24
  - The Egyptian Words and Symbols for the Mystery Teachings of YOGA 24
  - What is Egyptian Yoga? 24
    - The Term "Egyptian Yoga" and The Philosophy Behind It 24
- THE QUALITIES OF AN ASPIRANT 28
  - THE QUALIFICATIONS OF AN ASPIRANT 32
    - *QUESTION* 35
    - Good Association Part 1 36
- WHO IS A TEACHER 40
  - The Role of the Teacher 48
  - The key is in the _____ attitude with which you perform your duties 51
  - How to Approach a Spiritual Preceptor 52
    - The Concept of Sebai 58
- The Fundamental Principles of Neterian Religion 60
  - What is Neterianism and Who are the Neterians? 60
- Neterian Great Truths 62
  - The Great Truths of Neterianism are realized by means of Four Spiritual Disciplines in Three Steps 64
  - Summary of The Great Truths and the Shedy Paths to their Realization 66
- The Spiritual Culture and the Purpose of Life: Shetaut Neter 70
  - Shetaut Neter 70
  - Who is Neter in Kamitan Religion? 72
    - Sacred Scriptures of Shetaut Neter 72
- **SHETAUT ASAR-ASET-HERU** 72
- (C. 1580 B.C.E.-ROMAN PERIOD) 72
- (C. 3,000 B.C.E. – PTOLEMAIC PERIOD) 72
  - Neter and the Neteru 74

The Neteru 74
The Neteru and Their Temples 76
Listening to the Teachings 78
The Anunian Tradition 80
The Memphite Tradition 82
The Theban Tradition 84
The Goddess Tradition 86
The Asarian Tradition 88
The Aton Tradition 90
Akhnaton, Nefertiti and Daughters 90
The Great Awakening of Neterian Religion 92
The Teachings of the Temple of Isis and The Diet of the Initiates 94
The Recommended Daily Schedule for Yoga Practice 102
Basic Schedule of Spiritual Practice 104
Introduction to The Kemetic Yoga of Wisdom 106
Introduction to The Kemetic Yoga of Righteous Action 108
STEPS IN THE PRACTICE OF RIGHT ACTION YOGA 108
Ancient Egyptian Proverbs of 110
The Action Path 110
Introduction to the Kemetic Yoga of Postures and Movements 114
The Yogic Postures Discipline 116
Recreation: 118
Proper Breathing 120
Introduction to The Kemetic Yoga of Meditation 122
KAMITAN HISTORY – 5 MAIN STYLES OF MEDITATION DISCIPLINES - Shedy 122
Concentration - Meditation – Superconsciousness 122
Introduction to Meditation and Hekau 124
INTRODUCTION TO MEDITATION 124
When your body is _____ and you are thinking and feeling, you are mostly associated with your mind. What is Meditation? 127
Introduction to The Kemetic Yoga of Devotion 136
THE RELATIONSHIP BETWEEN RELIGION AND YOGA 140
How To Get Started On the Kemetic (Ancient Egyptian) Spiritual Path 142
WHAT IS THE NEXT STEP? 142
The Paths of Yoga 142
Integral Path: blending the disciplines to meet the needs of your personality 144
Setting Up The Personal Altar, To Practice The Daily Worship Program 154
Comportment and Demeanor As a Follower in the Spiritual Hall 160
Greeting the Spiritual Preceptor and The Term Seba 160
Sitting Postures 162
Respect for the Shrine and Conduct in the Temple 164
Spiritual Clothing 166
How to Overcome Failure on the Spiritual Path 168
The Spiritual Checklist 178
THE TRADITION OF INITIATION 182
The Ritual of Initiation 184

THE SEMA INSTITUTE AND TEMPLE OF SHETAUT NETER

Sema Institute of Yoga

Sema is an Ancient Egyptian word and symbol meaning union. The Sema Institute is dedicated to the propagation of the universal teachings of spiritual evolution which relate to the union of humanity and the union of all things within the universe. It is an organization that recognizes the unifying principles in all spiritual and religious systems of evolution throughout the world. Our primary goals are to provide the wisdom of ancient spiritual teachings from the Neterian Culture of Ancient Africa in books, courses and other forms of communication. The Institute is open to all who believe in the principles of peace, non-violence and spiritual emancipation regardless of sex, race, or creed. The Sema Institute is recognized by the United States of America Internal Revenue Service as a Nonprofit Spiritual Organization with 501(C3) status. All donations to the Sema Institute are tax deductible.

The Sema Institute and Temple of Shetaut Neter is dedicated to:

- ✓ **The dissemination of Neterian Wisdom (Sema and Shetaut Neter) in books,**
- ✓ **Neterianism is the modern day reference to Shetaut Neter (Ancient Egyptian Religion),**
- ✓ **Promoting the practice of Shetaut Neter Religion**
- ✓ **Training Neterian Aspirants,**
- ✓ **Promoting World Peace, human dignity and equality between cultures, genders and the care of the environment.**

PURPOSE OF THIS WORKBOOK: *This workbook helps by presenting the fundamental teachings of Egyptian Yoga and Neterian Spirituality with questions and exercises to help the aspirant gain a foundation for more advanced studies and practices*

AUTHOR Sebai Muata Ashby Ph. D., D.D., P.C., Y.U.

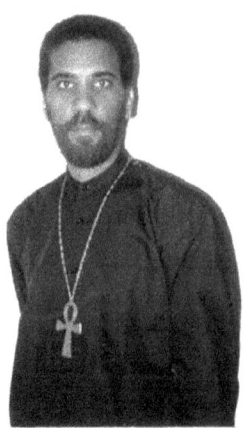

Sebai Muata Ashby was born in New York City but grew up in the Caribbean. Displaying an early interest in ancient civilizations and the Humanities, he began to study these subjects while in college but put these aside to work in the business world. After successfully running a business with his wife for several years they decided to pursue a deeper movement in life. Mr. Ashby began studies in the area of religion and philosophy and achieved doctorates in these areas while at the same time he began to collect his research into what would later become several books on the subject of the origins of Yoga Philosophy and practice in ancient Africa (Ancient Egypt) and also the origins of Christian Mysticism in Ancient Egypt. Muata Ashby discovered the vast philosophy of *Shetaut Neter* and *Sema* (Yoga mystical spirituality) practiced in ancient Africa and has written several book on this subject, detailing its history and practice for modern times. Muata Ashby also discovered the keys to understand the mystical code of the main traditions of Ancient Kamitan (Egyptian/African religion) known in ancient times as *Shetaut Neter*.

Muata Ashby holds a Doctor of Philosophy Degree in World Religion and Myth, focusing on African and Indian Religion, and a Doctor of Divinity Degree in Holistic Healing. He is also a Pastoral Counselor and Teacher of Yoga Philosophy and Discipline. Dr. Ashby received his Doctor of Divinity Degree from and is an adjunct faculty member of the American Institute of Holistic Theology and the Florida International University. Dr. Ashby is a certification as a PREP Relationship Counselor. Dr. Ashby has been an independent researcher and practitioner of Egyptian, Indian and Chinese Yoga and psychology as well as Christian Mysticism. Dr. Ashby has engaged in Post Graduate research in Yoga at the Yoga Research Foundation. He has extensively studied mystical religious traditions from around the world and is an accomplished lecturer, artist, poet, screenwriter, playwright and author of over 30 books on yoga and spiritual philosophy. He is an Ordained Minister and Spiritual Counselor and also the founder the Sema Institute, a non-profit organization dedicated to spreading the wisdom of Yoga and the Ancient Egyptian mystical traditions.

Dr. Muata Ashby has dedicated his life to educating all those interested in the mystical teachings of Yoga philosophy from Ancient Egypt. He conducts classes in Miami Florida on all aspects of Yoga wisdom and lifestyle.

Hemit Dja Un Nefert Ashby

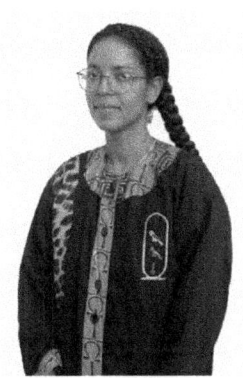

Hemit Dja Un Nefert Ashby, "Dja" is the spiritual partner of Dr. Muata Ashby. Seba Dja) was born in Guyana, South America, a heritage including African, Native American and European cultures. In 1975 her family moved to the United States. She is a Kamitan (Ancient Egyprian) priestess, initiate of the Temple Shetaut Neter-Aset (Egyptian Mysteries), Sema Tawi-Egyptian Yoga, and an independent researcher, practitioner and teacher of Sema (Smai) Tawi (Kamitan) and Indian Integral Yoga Systems, a Doctor of Veterinary Medicine, a Pastoral Spiritual Counselor, a Pastoral Health and Nutrition Counselor, and a Sema (Smai) Tawi Life-style Consultant." Dr. Ashby has engaged in post-graduate research in advanced Jnana, Bhakti, Karma, Raja and Kundalini Yogas at the Sema Institute of Yoga and Yoga Research Foundation, and has also worked extensively with her husband and spiritual partner, Dr. Muata Ashby, author of the Egyptian Yoga Book Series, editing many of these books, as well as studying, writing and lecturing in the area of Kamitan Yoga and Spirituality. She is a certified Tjef Neteru Sema Paut (Kamitan Yoga Exercise system) and Indian Hatha Yoga Exercise instructor, the Coordinator and Instructor for the Level 1 Teacher Certification Tjef Neteru Sema Training programs, and a teacher of health and stress management applications of the Yoga / Sema Tawi systems for modern society, based on the Kamitan and/or Indian yogic principles. Also, she is the co-author of "The Egyptian Yoga Exercise Workout Book," a contributing author for "The Kamitan Diet, Food for Body, Mind and Soul," author of the soon to be released, "Yoga Mystic Metaphors for Enlightenment."

INTRODUCTION

Udja and Greetings,
The Temple of Shetaut Neter in association with the Hemu of Shetaut Neter presents an "Introduction to Shetaut Neter"- Level 1. A 6 week course designed for the Rekhyt as well as the Shemsu. The purpose of this course is designed to offer a firm foundation in understanding Shetaut Neter also to serve as the first step through the initiatic system..
This course (Level 1) will have its own workbook all of which is derived from the 'Initiation into Egyptian Yoga'. Participants will each be required to have a workbook. Following this course, it will be immediately followed by a Level 2 class which will run for 4 weeks. This class is a pre-requisite for those requesting initiation.
For more information or questions please contact your local Hemu for any assistance needed. Hetep.

Sema Institute
Temple of Shetaut Neter.

A Brief History of Shetaut Neter

Early Beginnings: The First Religion

Ancient Egypt was the first and most ancient civilization to create a religious system that was complete with all three stages of religion, as well as an advanced spiritual philosophy of righteousness, called Maat Philosophy, that also had secular dimensions. Several temple systems were developed in Kamit; they were all related. The pre-Judaic/Islamic religions that the later Jewish and Muslim religions drew from in order to create their religions developed out of these, ironically enough, only to later repudiate the source from whence they originated. In any case, the Great Sphinx remains the oldest known religious monument in history that denotes high culture and civilization as well. Ancient Egypt and Nubia produced the oldest religious systems and their contact with the rest of the world led to the proliferation of advanced religion and spiritual philosophy. People who were practicing simple animism, shamanism, nature based religions and witchcraft were elevated to the level of not only understanding the nature of the Supreme Being, but also attaining salvation from the miseries of life through the effective discovery of that Transcendental being, not as an untouchable aloof Spirit, but as the very essence of all that exists.

NETERIANISM 10.000 B.C.E. – 2001 A.C.E.

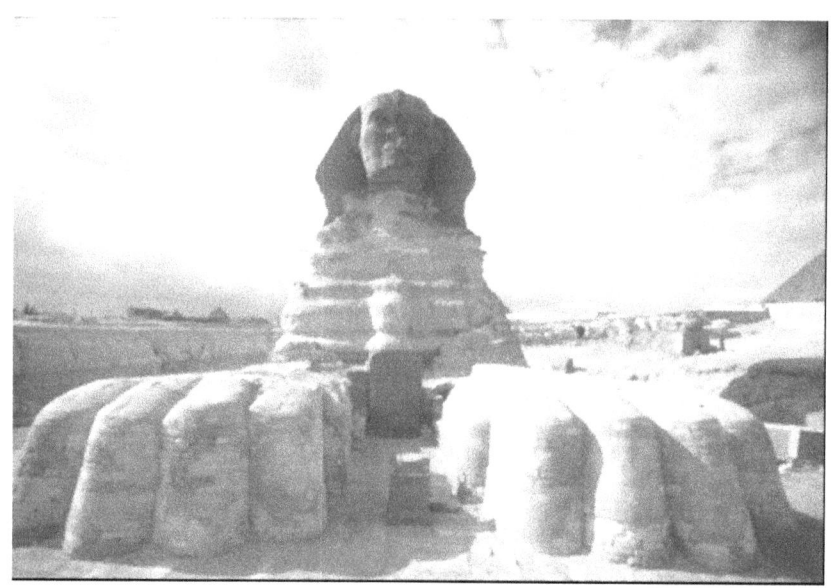

NOTES:

1. Week 1 Topic #2 Origin and Brief History.

Ancient Egypt and _____ produced the oldest _____ systems

The Term Kamit and the Origins of the Ancient Egyptians

The Ancient Egyptians recorded that they were originally a colony of Ethiopians from the south who came to the north east part of Africa. The term "Ethiopian," "Nubian," and "Kushite" all relate to the same peoples who lived south of Egypt. In modern times, the land which was once known as Nubia ("Land of Gold"), is currently known as the Sudan, and the land even further south and east towards the coast of east Africa is referred to as Ethiopia (see map above).

Recent research has shown that the modern Nubian word *kiji* means "fertile land, dark gray mud, silt, or black land." Since the sound of this word is close to the Ancient Egyptian name Kish or Kush, referring to the land south of Egypt, it is believed that the name Kush also meant "the land of dark silt" or "the black land." Kush was the Ancient Egyptian name for Nubia. Nubia, the black land, is the Sudan of today. Sudan is an Arabic translation of *sûd* which is the plural form of *aswad*, which means "black," and *ân* which means "of the." So, Sudan means "of the blacks." In the modern Nubian language, *nugud* means "black." Also, *nuger*, *nugur*, and *nubi* mean "black" as well. All of this indicates that the words Kush, Nubia, and Sudan all mean the same thing — the "black land" and/or the "land of the blacks."[1] As we will see, the differences between the term Kush and the term Kam (Qamit - name for Ancient Egypt in the Ancient Egyptian language) relate more to the same meaning but different geographical locations.

As we have seen, the terms "Ethiopia," "Nubia," "Kush" and "Sudan" all refer to "black land" and/or the "land of the blacks." In the same manner we find that the name of Egypt which was used by the Ancient Egyptians also means "black land" and/or the "land of the blacks." The hieroglyphs below reveal the Ancient Egyptian meaning of the words related to the name of their land. It is clear that the meaning of the word Qamit is equivalent to the word Kush as far as they relate to "black land" and that they also refer to a differentiation in geographical location, i.e. Kush is the "black land of the south" and Qamit is the "black land of the north." Both terms denote the primary quality that defines Africa, "black" or "Blackness" (referring to the land and its people). The quality of blackness and the consonantal sound of K or Q as well as the reference to the land are all aspects of commonality between the Ancient Kushitic and Kamitan terms.

The Hieroglyphic Text for the Name Qamit

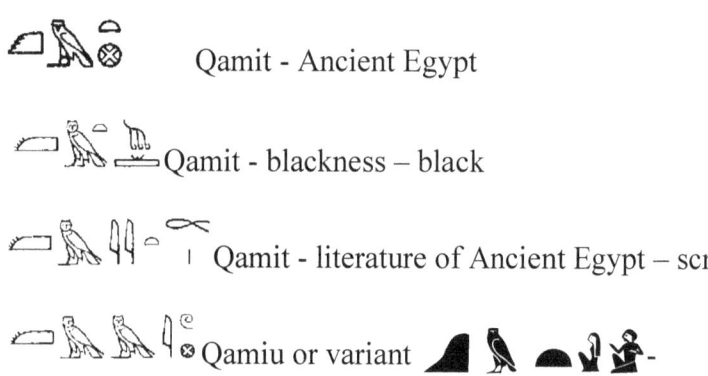

---

[1] "Nubia," *Microsoft® Encarta® Africana.* © 1999 Microsoft Corporation. All rights reserved.

QUESTION

What is the relationship between the Egyptians and Ethiopians?

NOTES:

Who Were the Ancient Egyptians and What is Yoga Philosophy?

The Ancient Egyptian religion (*Shetaut Neter*), language and symbols provide the first "historical" record of Yoga Philosophy and Religious literature. Egyptian Yoga is what has been commonly referred to by Egyptologists as Egyptian "Religion" or "Mythology", but to think of it as just another set of stories or allegories about a long lost civilization is to completely miss the greatest secret of human existence. Yoga, in all of its forms and disciplines of spiritual development, was practiced in Egypt earlier than anywhere else in history. This unique perspective from the highest philosophical system which developed in Africa over seven thousand years ago provides a new way to look at life, religion, the discipline of psychology and the way to spiritual development leading to spiritual Enlightenment. Egyptian mythology, when understood as a system of Yoga (union of the individual soul with the Universal Soul or Supreme Consciousness), gives every individual insight into their own divine nature and also a deeper insight into all religions and Yoga systems.

Diodorus Siculus (Greek Historian) writes in the time of Augustus (first century B.C.):

"Now the Ethiopians, as historians relate, were the first of all men and the proofs of this statement, they say, are manifest. For that they did not come into their land as immigrants from abroad but were the natives of it and so justly bear the name of autochthones (sprung from the soil itself), *is, they maintain, conceded by practically all men..."*

"They also say that the Egyptians are colonists sent out by the Ethiopians, Asar having been the leader of the colony. For, speaking generally, what is now Egypt, they maintain, was not land, but sea, when in the beginning the universe was being formed; afterwards, however, as the Nile during the times of its inundation carried down the mud from Ethiopia, land was gradually built up from the deposit...And the larger parts of the customs of the Egyptians are, they hold, Ethiopian, the colonists still preserving their ancient manners. For instance, the belief that their kings are Gods, the very special attention which they pay to their burials, and many other matters of a similar nature, are Ethiopian practices, while the shapes of their statues and the forms of their letters are Ethiopian; for of the two kinds of writing which the Egyptians have, that which is known as popular (demotic) *is learned by everyone, while that which is called sacred* (hieratic), *is understood only by the priests of the Egyptians, who learnt it from their Fathers as one of the things which are not divulged, but among the Ethiopians, everyone uses these forms of letters. Furthermore, the orders of the priests, they maintain, have much the same position among both peoples; for all are clean who are engaged in the service of the gods, keeping themselves shaven, like the Ethiopian priests, and having the same dress and form of staff, which is shaped like a plough and is carried by their kings who wear high felt hats which end in a knob in the top and are circled by the serpents which they call asps; and this symbol appears to carry the thought that it will be the lot who shall dare to attack the king to encounter death-carrying stings. Many other things are told by them concerning their own antiquity and the colony which they sent out that became the Egyptians, but about this there is no special need of our writing anything."*

The Ancient Egyptian texts state:

***"Our people originated at the base of the mountain of the Moon,
at the origin of the Nile river."***

"KMT"
"Egypt", "Burnt", "Land of Blackness","Land of the Burnt People."

NOTES:

Topic #3 Who were the Ancient Egyptian?

Many other things are told by them concerning their own antiquity and the colony which they sent out that became the _____,

Topic #4 What is Yoga Philosophy? A) Egyptian Religion

KMT (Ancient Egypt) is situated close to Lake Victoria in present day Africa. This is the same location where the earliest human remains have been found, in the land currently known as Ethiopia-Tanzania. Recent genetic technology as reported in the new encyclopedias and leading news publications has revealed that all peoples of the world originated in Africa and migrated to other parts of the world prior to the last Ice Age 40,000 years ago. Therefore, as of this time, genetic testing has revealed that all humans are alike. The earliest bone fossils which have been found in many parts of the world were those of the African Grimaldi type. During the Ice Age, it was not possible to communicate or to migrate. Those trapped in specific locations were subject to the regional forces of weather and climate. Less warmer climates required less body pigment, thereby producing lighter pigmented people who now differed from their dark-skinned ancestors. After the Ice Age when travel was possible, these light-skinned people who had lived in the northern, colder regions of harsh weather during the Ice Age period moved back to the warmer climates of their ancestors, and mixed with the people there who had remained dark-skinned, thereby producing the Semitic colored people. "Semite" means mixture of skin color shades.

Therefore, there is only one human race who, due to different climactic and regional exposure, changed to a point where there seemed to be different "types" of people. Differences were noted with respect to skin color, hair texture, customs, languages, and with respect to the essential nature (psychological and emotional makeup) due to the experiences each group had to face and overcome in order to survive.

From a philosophical standpoint, the question as to the origin of humanity is redundant when it is understood that _ALL_ come from one origin which some choose to call the "Big Bang" and others "The Supreme Being."

> **"Thou makest the color of the skin of one race to be different from that of another, but however many may be the varieties of mankind, it is thou that makes them all to live."**
> —Ancient Egyptian Proverb from *The Hymns of Amun*

> **"Souls, Heru, son, are of the self-same nature, since they came from the same place where the Creator modeled them; nor male nor female are they. Sex is a thing of bodies not of Souls."**
> —Ancient Egyptian Proverb from *The teachings of Aset to Heru*

Historical evidence proves that Ethiopia-Nubia already had Kingdoms at least 300 years before the first Kingdom-Pharaoh of Egypt.

> *"Ancient Egypt was a colony of Nubia - Ethiopia. ...Asar having been the leader of the colony..."*

> *"And upon his return to Greece, they gathered around and asked, "tell us about this great land of the Blacks called Ethiopia." And Herodotus said, "There are two great Ethiopian nations, one in Sind (India) and the other in Egypt."*

> **Recorded by Egyptian high priest *Manetho* (300 B.C.)**
> **also Recorded by *Diodorus* (Greek historian 100 B.C.)**

The pyramids themselves however, cannot be dated, but indications are that they existed far back in antiquity. The Pyramid Texts (hieroglyphics inscribed on pyramid walls) and Coffin Texts (hieroglyphics inscribed on coffins) speak authoritatively on the constitution of the human spirit, the vital Life Force along the human spinal cord (known in India as *"Kundalini"*), the immortality of the soul, reincarnation and the law of Cause and Effect (known in India as the Law of Karma).

QUESTION

Those trapped in specific locations were subject to the regional forces of _____ and _____.

NOTES:

What is Initiation?

What does it mean to tread the spiritual path of Kemetic Yoga? Being an initiate is not what most people think of when they hear of a yoga practitioner. There are many misconceptions about the teachings of yoga and there are many misconceptions about those who practice yoga. Sometimes the image of a cross-legged man with matted locks comes to mind. Sometimes wandering ascetics come to mind. Sometimes an image of an incredibly limber person in some impossible posture comes to mind. Sometimes a figure in a meditation posture transcending the world comes to mind. Also sometimes people think that yoga can drive you crazy so they picture a fanatical person uttering intelligible words. Sometimes the image of the media and from the traditional church has promoted an image of occult, mysterious and unnatural personalities as practitioners of yoga so they also picture cults and fanaticism.

What is Initiation? The great personalities of the past known to the world as Isis, Hathor, Jesus, Buddha and many other great Sages and Saints were initiated into their spiritual path but how did initiation help them and what were they specifically initiated into?

Many people think of initiation, when associated with spiritual studies, as some kind of fantastic event which will in and of itself cause a major transformation in a person's life. Initiation should be thought of less as an event and more as the process of embarking on a journey of spiritual living which will lead to spiritual enlightenment. With this broad understanding it should be clear that this entire book is initiating you, the reader, into the higher teachings of life. Every time you turn a page you are learning more and more about the world and as you do you are learning more about yourself. In this section we will discuss the process of initiation and the way in which spiritual knowledge is imparted. This volume is a template for such lofty studies, a guidebook and blueprint for aspirants who want to understand what the path is all about, its requirements and goals, as they work with a qualified spiritual guide as they tread the path of Kemetic Spirituality and Yoga disciplines.

From time immemorial the tradition of teacher and student has been carried on by Sages and Saints the world over. This is evident even in the world religions. Hetheru of Ancient Egypt was initiated by Djehuty. Heru (Horus) of Ancient Egypt was initiated into the mystical teachings by Aset (Isis). Rama (a form of Krishna from India) was initiated into the teachings by Sage Vasistha. Jesus was initiated into the teachings by John the Baptist. As in any other discipline of life spiritual studies require an authentic teacher. However, even the greatest teacher cannot teach a person who is not qualified to learn. Therefore, we will begin by enumerating the ten virtues of a spiritual aspirant. These imply the qualities that anyone desiring to practice spirituality needs to work on to develop.

The teachings of Yoga and Mystical religion are the means by which an ordinary human being can rise to the state of spiritual enlightenment, inner fulfillment, peace and abiding happiness in life. These teachings were in ancient times passed on through an exact system which involves listening to, study of and meditation upon the teachings in a proper environment and with proper guidance. This method of teaching is known as *Initiatic Way of Education.* There are many styles of Yoga, although their goals are all the same: Union with the divine. These include: Yoga of Intuitive Wisdom of the Divine, Yoga of Devotional Union with the Divine, Yoga of Meditation and Mind Control, Yoga of Virtuous Living, Yoga of Cultivation of the Latent Life Force Energy (Serpent Power).

The Initiatic Way of Education

Yoga philosophy originated at the dawn of civilization in the present era of human history beginning with the emergence of the Ancient Egyptian civilization. The temple system provided a unique format for education and government which was able to sustain and provide for the needs of Ancient Egypt for over 5,000 years. Therefore, it is useful here to briefly describe the Temple System of education and a method in which its wisdom can be applied to modern society.

NOTES:

Topic #6 What is Initiation?

Initiation is more of an embarking on a journey of……………………………………….which leads to spiritual……………………………..

Since the teachings of yoga and mystical spirituality have been traditionally passed on through the teacher-student relationship for over two millennia, this system of education is integral to the study of transpersonal disciplines. While in modern times the local parish priest, the counselor or psychotherapist have taken the place of the Sages, they have not adopted the wisdom nor the ancient method of education employed by their forebears. Thus the *Guru-disciple relationship* and the *Initiatic way of education* are important areas of study for the aspiring Transpersonal Studies student or professional.

The need for a true teacher of spirituality cannot be overemphasized in the course of spiritual practice. This is the reason why so many "new age" teachers and even members of the traditional establishment have gone to "sit at the feet," so to speak, of Eastern teachers of yoga and mystical philosophy. This is also the reason why much of the research done by early transpersonal researchers, beginning with Carl Jung, focuses on the Initiatic relationship, as well as the wisdom which is imparted through it. An aspirant is like an athlete. He or she needs coaching and practice in order to attain mastery over the lower nature. In every area of your life where you have achieved success, it is because you studied and practiced, if not in this lifetime, in a previous one. Spiritual Enlightenment cannot be achieved through magic or through unnatural means. It is achieved through understanding and hard work, not ordinary work, but those activities which lead to purification of the heart.

It is possible to promote spiritual growth through the books written by genuine spiritual preceptors. The new forms of media such as audio and video have gone even further in conveying the message of the teachings to the entire world. However, at some point, books and tapes can only go so far in explaining the fruits of the true practice of spirituality. This is because the mind can develop many misconceptions and illusions about spirituality just as in any area of ordinary worldly life. Therefore, a guide or coach who is advanced in its practice should be sought out and approached with humility and honesty to ask questions and dispel subtle forms of ignorance. This is the process of spiritual teaching called Initiation. The aspirant is initiated into a philosophy and way of life which he or she needs to learn and practice by studying, reflecting and meditating on the teachings. Initiation is a conscious choice to adopt a teaching and to embark on the task of basing one's life on it in order to purify one's mind and body through the teaching, so that one may become a conduit of transcendental forms of experience.

One of the main problems of society is the relative lack of interest in the scriptures and secondly, the relatively small number of authentic spiritual preceptors available to teach those who are interested. Many people do not find spirituality attractive because they feel they would "lose" out on life if they became seriously involved. Others see the prospect of spirituality as being too remote for their understanding.

An authentic Spiritual Preceptor is not only someone who is advanced on the spiritual path, or even just someone who has reached the fully enlightened state. A Guru, in the Upanishadic (teachings of the Indian Upanishads) sense of the word, is someone who is spiritually enlightened and who also is well versed in the scriptural teachings and methods of training aspirants according to their level of understanding. Therefore, a Sehu or counselor of Kemetic Yoga must first achieve a high degree of understanding and personal - spiritual emancipation since the subtleties of the mind must be well understood. The teacher must be able to be a refuge for all people, have an extensive knowledge of the teachings pertaining to his/her level of attainment, and enthusiastically pursue all forms of Yoga.

Every true mystical tradition, be it religious or non-religious, requires a traditional link because the Initiatic teaching given to those who become initiated into a tradition, needs the benefit of a preceptor who has received the teaching from a previously initiated teacher and has correct understanding of the teaching. Otherwise it would be, as an Eastern parable explains, like a blind person trying to explain to other blind people what the world looks like simply using imagination and wit. There are others, intellectuals, who come to believe that they have attained "Enlightenment" because they read the scriptures. However, upon being tested in the world of human experience, the complexes and sufferings of life resurface. Thus, a need for a comprehensive program of spiritual development is necessary to promote real and abiding transformation in the human heart.

QUESTION

How does the Kemetic Yoga counselor help the seeker?

How should a beginning spiritual aspirant think about the different levels of aspirants?

In the beginning, the Kemetic (Egyptian) Yogic Teacher helps the individual to somehow turn the anguish, disappointment and pain experienced as a result of interaction with the world into a desire to rise above it, as symbolized by the lotus rising out of the muddy waters. To this end, a series of techniques and disciplines have been developed over thousands of years. The Sehu or Kemetic Yoga counselor needs to help the seeker restructure and channel those energies which arise from disappointment and frustration into a healthy dispassion of the world and its entanglements, spiritual aspiration and self-effort directed at sustaining a viable personal spiritual program or *Sheti(also written as Shedy)*. In the *Shetaut Neter* system of yoga from Ancient Egypt or Egyptian Yoga, there were three levels of aspirants.

1- ASPIRATION- Students who are being instructed on a probationary status, and have not experienced inner vision. The important factor at this level is ***awakening of the Spiritual Self,*** that is, becoming conscious of the divine presence within one's self and the universe by having faith that there is a spiritual essence beyond ordinary human understanding.

2- STRIVING- Students who have attained inner vision and have received a glimpse of cosmic consciousness. The important factor at this level is ***purgation of the self,*** that is, purification of mind and body through a spiritual discipline. The aspirant tries to totally surrender "personal" identity or ego to the divine inner Self which is the Universal Self of all Creation.

3- ESTABLISHED- Students who have become IDENTIFIED with or UNITED with GOD. The important factor at this level is ***illumination of the intellect,*** that is, experience and appreciation of the divine presence during reflection and meditation, <u>Union</u> with the divine self, the divine marriage of the individual with the universal.

In order to have a better understanding of what initiation is we must look into the distant past in order to discover its purpose and use.

In the *Shetaut Neter* system of yoga from Ancient Egypt or Egyptian Yoga, there were _____ levels of aspirants.

PERSONAL ASSESSMENT

Before proceeding with the book any further, it is important that you assess yourself so that you may begin to reflect on your current status in terms of your position in life as well as your spiritual evolution. Answer the following questions and keep them for your own record. They will serve you by helping you to understand what you feel at the present time and what direction you want your life to take.

1- How would you describe your knowledge of religion and philosophy?

2- What do you see as the greatest obstacle to your happiness and fulfillment in life?

3- What do you see as the most important need that you have?

4- What is your previous religious affiliation or faith and how do you think that relates to what you are following now?

5- What role do you feel religion or spirituality plays in your life?

6- Have you had any previous Yoga instruction? If so where and what was (is) your experience?

7- Have you received any advanced religious instruction?

8- How do you see your life?

9- What do you think of your own potential to succeed in life?

10- If you could, what would you like to do with your life?

Answer the personal assessment Questions:

Yoga in Ancient Egypt

The Egyptian Words and Symbols for the Mystery Teachings of YOGA

The first and most important teaching to understand in our study surrounds the Ancient Egyptian word "Shedy." Shedy comes from the root "Sheta." The Ancient Egyptian word *Sheta* means something which is *hidden, secret, unknown*, or *cannot be seen through or understood, a secret, a mystery*. What is considered to be inert matter also possesses *Hidden Properties or Shetau Akhet*. Rituals, Words of Power (Khu-Hekau, Mantras), religious texts and pictures are S*hetaut Neter* or *Divine Mysteries. Shetat* or *Seshetat* are the secret rituals in the cults of the Egyptian Gods. *Shetai* is the *Hidden God, incomprehensible God, Mysterious One, Secret One*. One name of the soul of Amun is *Shet-ba* (The One whose soul is hidden). The name Amun itself signifies "The Hidden One": *Shetai. Shedy* (spiritual discipline) is to go deeply into the mysteries, to study the mystery teachings and literature profoundly, to penetrate the mysteries. *Nehas-t* signifies: "resurrection" or "spiritual awakening." The body or *Shet-t* (mummy) is where a human being can focuses attention to practice spiritual disciplines. When spiritual discipline is perfected the true self or *Shti* (he who is hidden in the coffin) is revealed.

Thus, Shedy is the spiritual discipline or program to promote spiritual evolution which was used in Ancient Egypt. Now we can begin to discover the teachings of that spiritual program. These all fall under the broad term "Egyptian Yoga."

What is Egyptian Yoga?

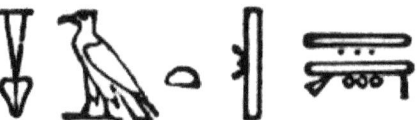

Smai Tawi
(From Chapter 4 of
the *Prt m Hru*)

The Term "Egyptian Yoga" and The Philosophy Behind It

As previously discussed, Yoga in all of its forms were practiced in Egypt apparently earlier than anywhere else in our history. This point of view is supported by the fact that there is documented scriptural and iconographical evidence of the disciplines of virtuous living, dietary purification, study of the wisdom teachings and their practice in daily life, psychophysical and psycho-spiritual exercises and meditation being practiced in Ancient Egypt, long before the evidence of its existence is detected in India (including the Indus Valley Civilization) or any other early civilization (Sumer, Greece, China, etc.).

The teachings of Yoga are at the heart of *Prt m Hru*. As explained earlier, the word "Yoga" is a Sanskrit term meaning to unite the individual with the Cosmic. The term has been used in certain parts of this book for ease of communication since the word "Yoga" has received wide popularity especially in western countries in recent years. The Ancient Egyptian equivalent term to the Sanskrit word yoga is: **"Smai."** **Smai** means union, and the following determinative terms give it a spiritual significance, at once equating it with the term "Yoga"

NOTES:

Week 2 Topic#1: Yoga in Ancient Egypt?

_____ is the spiritual discipline or program to promote spiritual _____ which was used in Ancient Egypt as it is used in India. When used in conjunction with the Ancient Egyptian symbol which means land, ***"Ta,"*** the term "union of the two lands" arises.

In Chapter 4 and Chapter 17 of the *Prt m Hru,* a term "Smai Tawi" is used. It means "Union of the two lands of Egypt," ergo "Egyptian Yoga." The two lands refer to the two main districts of the country (North and South). In ancient times, Egypt was divided into two sections or land areas. These were known as Lower and Upper Egypt. In Ancient Egyptian mystical philosophy, the land of Upper Egypt relates to the divinity Heru (Heru (Horus)), who represents the Higher Self, and the land of Lower Egypt relates to Set, the divinity of the lower self. So ***Smai Taui*** means "the union of the two lands" or the "Union of the lower self with the Higher Self. The lower self relates to that which is negative and uncontrolled in the human mind including worldliness, egoism, ignorance, etc. (Set), while the Higher Self relates to that which is above temptations and is good in the human heart as well as in touch with transcendental consciousness (Heru). Thus, we also have the Ancient Egyptian term ***Smai Heru-Set,*** or the union of Heru and Set. So Smai Taui or Smai Heru-Set are the Ancient Egyptian words which are to be translated as "**Egyptian Yoga.**"

Above: the main symbol of Egyptian Yoga: *Sma.* The Ancient Egyptian language and symbols provide the first "historical" record of Yoga Philosophy and Religious literature. The hieroglyph Sma, "Sema," represented by the union of two lungs and the trachea, symbolizes that the union of the duality, that is, the Higher Self and lower self, leads to Non-duality, the One, singular consciousness.

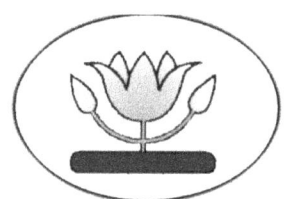

Question

Topic #2: What is Egyptian Yoga?

The term............................or......................................are Ancient Egyptian words which are to translated as Egyptian Yoga

THE QUALITIES OF AN ASPIRANT

The first qualification necessary for a spiritual aspirant is that he or she must have the *initiative* or primary interest in advancing spiritually. It is no coincidence that the word "initiative" and the word "initiation" convey a similar connotation. You must be the one to take the first step toward your own spiritual emancipation. You must be the one to approach others of higher spiritual development so that you may begin to discover the path which you wish to follow toward your eventual freedom from all worldly pains and sorrows. In short, it is you who must put forth the effort which will affect your own liberation from the bondage of illusion and ignorance which grips the masses of people all over the world. Having discovered this initiative within yourself, you are qualified to receive spiritual instruction.

The ancient spiritual texts of all traditions state that it behooves an aspirant to seek out the true wisdom which alleviates the pain and sorrow of human existence while elevating the human spirit. If the wisdom one holds has not produced an improvement in one's quality of life, then it is possible that the teaching or its practice is wrong. In the task of spiritual practice there is no mediator between oneself and one's higher Self. However, a guide is needed to show the way to discover the true Self in much the same way as any other human endeavor. Someone who is knowledgeable about the spiritual path can help in advising and teaching others. Take for example a concert pianist or an N.B.A. basketball star. Both of these professionals perfected their skills through correct teaching and practice, beginning from a point of utter ignorance to the level of spontaneous performance. In order to excel at spiritual development, one must apply the correct technique and practice daily. This is the path of Yoga, exercising conscious effort every day to unite oneself with the higher Self.

Yoga, the union of the individual human consciousness with the universal consciousness, can occur without any special instruction from a religious or a spiritual preceptor. This is known as the path of nature or as it is better known, the school of hard knocks. It involves repeated incarnations, pain and suffering, to teach you the futility of trying to find abiding happiness in the world rather than within yourself.

Although much of the Egyptian teachings have diffused into the world religions, in the course of time they have been misinterpreted and reconfigured so that there is great confusion and misunderstanding as to their true meaning. This has created a situation in which many present day clergy speak the teachings but do not have a clear understanding of how to apply them in their own lives to transcend the pain and suffering of existence, let alone, be able to enlighten their followers as to how to evolve spiritually.

Yoga is a tradition which has established a long proven record of success in teaching those who desire to discover the Self. The traditional approach to yoga instruction has been broken up into three stages. These are: 1-Listening, 2-Reflection and 3- Meditation. In a broad sense, you will be instructed in this same manner throughout this book series. First you will receive the teaching, then you will be assisted in reflecting on that teaching and incorporating it into your life. You will then be instructed on how to intensify your reflective movement and gradually reach a meditative state of concentration on the divine.

Every true mystical tradition, be it religious or non-religious, requires a traditional mystical link because initiatic teaching given to those who become initiated into a tradition, needs the benefit of a preceptor who has received the teaching from an enlightened teacher and has correct understanding of the teaching. Otherwise it would be, as an Eastern parable explains, like a blind person trying to explain to other blind people what the world looks like simply using imagination and wit. There are others, intellectuals, who come to believe that they have attained "Enlightenment" because they read the scriptures. However, when they are tested by natural human situations of adversity, they cannot control their emotions or find mental peace. Some, immersed in the subtle ignorance and egoism of the mind don't even realize their misunderstanding of the teachings and of their own attainment or spiritual level.

NOTES:

Topic: The Qualities of an Aspirant?

Aspirant must have the primary……………………….in advancing spiritually

What is the path of nature and in light of that, **how should a spiritual aspirant think about their spiritual path**?

Others study the teachings with earnestness and great seriousness and find that they cannot realize the subtlety of the teachings in order to effect their Enlightenment. They find that they cannot control their minds, emotions or desires as the teachings suggest and thus are unable to discover the deeper meaning of the teachings.

An example of the inability to control the mind is the cigarette smoker. He or she "knows" that smoking is poisonous and yet they are unable to stop. Why? Because their self-knowledge is superficial (egoistic) and they have not discovered the wellspring of will and inner fulfillment within themselves so they continue to search for fulfillment outside of themselves through objects which seem to gratify their needs. In reality, these external habits that seem to bring pleasure are in reality leading to greater pain and disappointment. i.e. asthma, heart disease and lung cancer along with greater restlessness and mental unrest.

Still, others seek to escape the world as they know it by immersing themselves in work, drugs or other intense distractions. An example of this type of personality is someone who needs constant activity so as not to feel lonely or bored. This personality is constantly searching for action by turning on the television, calling someone, gossiping or having some other interaction. If this attitude becomes intensified, this personality seeks to agitate him/herself constantly by always finding something to be upset or argumentative about. Unless there is a fight or other intense emotion present, this personality feels lost. Those who suffer from this defect have developed an intense dependency on sense perceptions and emotions. They cannot feel right unless there is some activity present, be it positive or negative. Even if there is no trouble, they will create trouble, so as to agitate their minds and feel "alive."

A sage does not live a life based on the sense perceptions nor on the desires of the mind and body. He or she has discovered the illusoriness of the senses, the emptiness of desires and the futility of trying to fulfill them in the realm of time and space. Those who are advancing on the spiritual path have discovered that they do not need to lean on sense perceptions to feel alive, nor on events to make themselves feel happy. They have begun to discover that sustenance and happiness comes from within. It is there that all desires are truly fulfilled. For this reason, proper initiation into a teaching and learning under the instruction of an enlightened master or a senior student who is in association with a master is necessary in order to develop the correct understanding and practice of the teachings.

While the teachings may seem explicit to the highly intellectual mind, there are nuances of misunderstanding which will occur. This is why association with an authentic teacher is essential on the spiritual path for those who are serious about their spiritual development. Any other learning process is subject to error and confusion which will lead to disappointment and frustration. The initiatic teachings exist as an alternative to ordinary worldly thinking.

Christianity, having originally been an initiatic mystery religion, was no different in its approach of the transference of the teachings from teacher to student. Long before the establishment of Christianity as a religion, water was used in ceremonies to initiate new followers into the philosophy of mystery religions. Prior to entering a temple in Egypt and other countries, people would bathe as a symbol of inner purification. Christianity adopted this ritual and it was used at the initiation of Jesus by John the Baptist. This ritual act served to link Jesus to a tradition into which he would later initiate his disciples as well. But what was this initiatic relationship all about? What was its purpose and how was this purpose to be accomplished? These are very important questions for anyone seriously considering treading the spiritual path. Therefore, it is appropriate here to discuss what aspiration really means and what an authentic teacher is.

QUESTION

A sage does not live a life based on the _____ perceptions nor on the desires of the mind and body

NOTES:

THE QUALIFICATIONS OF AN ASPIRANT

"When the student is ready, the master will appear."

"Those who understand or believe will be persecuted and ridiculed."

—Ancient Egyptian Proverbs

When a person begins to wonder about the origin of the universe, the purpose of life, the cruelty of life, the inability to be truly happy in the world and the transitoriness of all things, such a person may be ready to inquire about the deeper truths of her/his own existence and to seek answers to such questions which have plagued them for perhaps many lifetimes.

The reason that most people accept the injustices, cruelties and sorrows of the world is that they tend to overlook the obvious illusoriness of relationships and the fleeting nature of sensory pleasure. There is lack of inquiry into the nature of pain so people go on believing that they will eventually find happiness in the world. They believe that pain is just a "normal" part of human life and as such must be accepted and dealt with as best as possible when it occurs or that they just need to be more careful to avoid painful situations in the future. They almost never entertain questions about the unreality of the world and life in general and when they do, they might turn to others who are as intensely involved in the world and by so doing, become once again distracted with the burdens of life.

"Passions and irrational desires are ills exceedingly great; and over these GOD hath set up the Mind to play the part of judge and executioner."

—Ancient Egyptian Proverb

A spiritual aspirant or initiate may be defined as: anyone seriously seeking spiritual development and chooses to enter (be initiated) into a lifestyle directed toward spiritual realization rather than perishable worldly attainments. But what is this lifestyle? What is required to make the goals of spiritual life become reality? Who is qualified to practice yoga and what does it mean to be a serious yogi(ni)?

People who have trouble coping with life sometimes seek help through counseling with psychologists, priests, pastoral counselors or friends. In the case of a Yoga counselor or a Yogic Spiritual Preceptor, the benefits of such an association are a step beyond those of ordinary psychology and psychotherapy which seek to integrate one's personality into the accepted "norms" of the mainstream society and which considers anyone who does not adhere to such standards to be abnormal. From the perspective of yoga philosophy, much of the accepted "normal" behavior is really insane behavior which has been accepted as "normal." For example, it is accepted as "normal" to gossip, to use profanity, to become angry at others, up to a point. It is all right to scream at someone, but if you hit them then you could be sued. When that point is crossed, then measures are taken by society in an attempt to curb such behavior. In this sense, the mind of the ordinary human being is conditioned by what society promotes and what the desires and thoughts in the mind compel the person to do. From this perspective of what most people have come to know and for the most part, accept as "normal" human behavior, yoga pushes the aspirant to become "super normal." It pushes the aspirant to rise beyond his/her current level of so-called "normal" mental conditioning to conquer anger, hatred, greed, impatience, sadness, discontent and the improper use of words within him/herself.

"When emotions are societies objective, tyranny will govern regardless of the ruling class."

"Indulge not thyself in the passion of Anger; it is whetting a sword to wound thine own breast, or murder thy friend."

—Ancient Egyptian Proverbs

NOTES:

Topic Qualification of an Aspirant?

From the perspective of yoga philosophy, much of the accepted "_____" behavior is really insane behavior which has been accepted as "_____."

Yoga is a process of reversing the conditioning effect which ordinary human life has on the mind. Everything which affects the mind conditions the mind; this is the nature of the mind. Ignorance of the Self is the primary and most important concern in yoga because ordinary human life intensifies ignorance, and thereby human pain and suffering as well. Yoga un-conditions the mind in order that the aspirant may attain unity with his/her Higher Self and achieve supreme freedom and supreme peace in the state of Heru (Horus)hood (Godhood, Christhood or Kingdom of Heaven, Liberation, Moksha, Enlightenment), instead of being trapped in the confines of the ego-self. In this sense, the practice of yoga conditions the mind so it experiences expansion while worldly conditioning and egoism results in mental contraction, dependency on the world and intensification of pain and suffering.

In the beginning, the Yogic Counselor must help the individual to somehow turn the anguish and pain experienced as a result of interaction with the world, into a desire to rise above it, as symbolized by the lotus rising out of the waters. To this end, a series of techniques and disciplines have been developed over thousands of years. The Yoga counselor needs to help the seeker restructure and channel those energies which arise from disappointment and frustration into a healthy dispassion of the world and its entanglements and spiritual aspiration and self-effort directed at sustaining a viable personal spiritual program or *Sadhana*.

The ancient Egyptian Mystery system is called *Shetaut NETER* meaning the knowledge of the hidden or secret (Shetaut) way of the Gods and Goddesses (*NETER*). Shetaut is also the name of the Absolute, the hidden and transcendental Supreme Being which sustains creation and is synonymous with the terms or names *Amun* and *Nebertcher*. In the *Shetaut NETER* system of yoga, there were three levels of aspirants.

1- **The Mortals**: Students who were being instructed on a probationary status, but had not experienced inner vision.

2- **The Intelligences**: Students who had attained inner vision and had received a glimpse of cosmic consciousness.

3- **The Creators or Beings of Light:** Students who had become IDENTIFIED with or UNITED with the light (GOD).

The teachings surrounding the cult of ISIS give important information concerning the conduct necessary to be an initiate in the mysteries of spiritual development (YOGA). The *Veil of Isis* is the veil of ignorance which blocks divine awareness from human perception. The following teaching reveals the nature of Isis, who in this aspect represents the all-encompassing Divine Self.

"I Isis, am all that has been, all that is, or shall be;
and no mortal man hath ever unveiled me."

NOTES:

Topic Qualification of an Aspirant?

From the perspective of yoga philosophy, much of the accepted "_____" behavior is really insane behavior which has been accepted as "_____."

Yoga is a process of reversing the conditioning effect which ordinary human life has on the mind. Everything which affects the mind conditions the mind; this is the nature of the mind. Ignorance of the Self is the primary and most important concern in yoga because ordinary human life intensifies ignorance, and thereby human pain and suffering as well. Yoga un-conditions the mind in order that the aspirant may attain unity with his/her Higher Self and achieve supreme freedom and supreme peace in the state of Heru (Horus)hood (Godhood, Christhood or Kingdom of Heaven, Liberation, Moksha, Enlightenment), instead of being trapped in the confines of the ego-self. In this sense, the practice of yoga conditions the mind so it experiences expansion while worldly conditioning and egoism results in mental contraction, dependency on the world and intensification of pain and suffering.

In the beginning, the Yogic Counselor must help the individual to somehow turn the anguish and pain experienced as a result of interaction with the world, into a desire to rise above it, as symbolized by the lotus rising out of the waters. To this end, a series of techniques and disciplines have been developed over thousands of years. The Yoga counselor needs to help the seeker restructure and channel those energies which arise from disappointment and frustration into a healthy dispassion of the world and its entanglements and spiritual aspiration and self-effort directed at sustaining a viable personal spiritual program or *Sadhana*.

The ancient Egyptian Mystery system is called *Shetaut NETER* meaning the knowledge of the hidden or secret (Shetaut) way of the Gods and Goddesses (*NETER*). Shetaut is also the name of the Absolute, the hidden and transcendental Supreme Being which sustains creation and is synonymous with the terms or names *Amun* and *Nebertcher*. In the *Shetaut NETER* system of yoga, there were three levels of aspirants.

1- **The Mortals**: Students who were being instructed on a probationary status, but had not experienced inner vision.

2- **The Intelligences**: Students who had attained inner vision and had received a glimpse of cosmic consciousness.

3- **The Creators or Beings of Light:** Students who had become IDENTIFIED with or UNITED with the light (GOD).

The teachings surrounding the cult of ISIS give important information concerning the conduct necessary to be an initiate in the mysteries of spiritual development (YOGA). The *Veil of Isis* is the veil of ignorance which blocks divine awareness from human perception. The following teaching reveals the nature of Isis, who in this aspect represents the all-encompassing Divine Self.

"I Isis, am all that has been, all that is, or shall be;
and no mortal man hath ever unveiled me."

QUESTION

The practice of yoga conditions the _____.

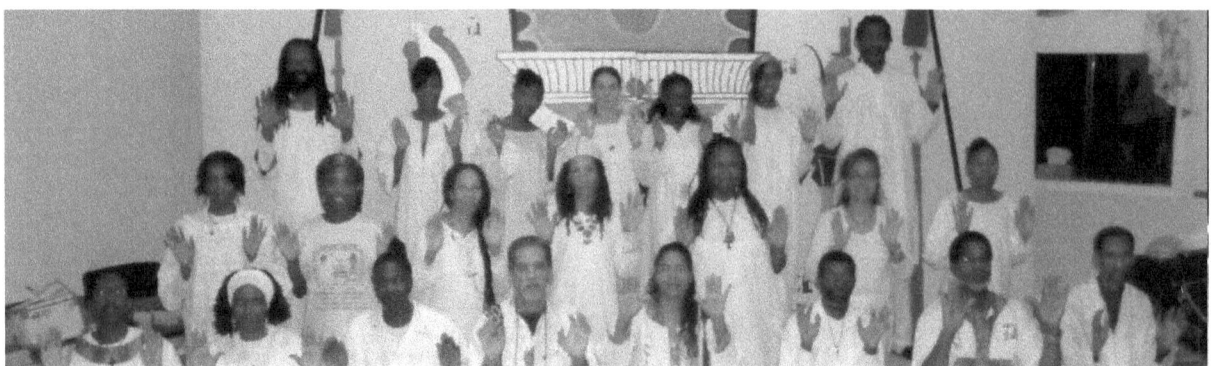

Good Association Part 1

One of the most important ways of promoting awareness and constant reflection is keeping the company of wise teachers or Sages. In ancient Egypt, the Temple system served the purpose of instructing aspirants in the wisdom teachings and then allowing them back into the world on a regular basis in order to test their level of understanding and self-control by practicing the teachings when confronted with ordinary, worldly minded people. The Temple was a place where the initiate could go on a regular basis to receive instruction and counseling on the correct application of the teachings in day to day life. The idea is reflected in the *Stela of Djehuty-Nefer*:

"Consume pure foods and pure thoughts with pure hands, adore celestial beings, become associated with wise ones: sages, saints and prophets; make offerings to GOD..."

The association with Sages and Saints (Good Association) is seen as a primary way to accelerate the spiritual development of the aspirant. Again, this is because it is the nature of the mind to imitate that which it focuses on. An important definition of the symbols associated with *Sma* 𓌻 or Sema is *to render clear or visible* 𓌻𓃀𓏏𓁹. In ancient Egypt, the *gathering, assembly or reunion* was called *Smait* 𓌻𓃀𓏏𓊖 and *Smai* 𓌻𓃀𓏥 is a name for the Temple, the gathering place. In Egypt, the priest assumed the role of preceptor, *Sbai* 𓀀𓊹𓏥𓉐𓃀, leading the initiate to understand the teachings of the hieroglyphs, to purification of the mind and body and eventually to intuitional realization through the practice of mental exercises and the application of the wisdom teachings. In ancient hieroglyphics, this is symbolized by the scenes where deities such as *Heru (Horus), Djehuty, Anubis, Hathor, Isis*, etc. lead the initiate to meet Osiris (his/her Higher Self). In India, this process is known as *"Satsanga"* where the aspirant receives teaching from the *Guru* (Spiritual Preceptor) on a continuous basis. In Buddhism the process is known as *Sanga*. In Christianity this idea was reflected in the relationship between Jesus and John the Baptist and later between Jesus and his disciples. Keeping the company of wise ones is an important and powerful tool for spiritual development because the nature of the unenlightened (ignorant) mind allows it to make subtle mistakes which can lead the aspirant astray from the correct interpretation of the teachings. Thus, receiving the teaching is the real force which causes transformation through a baptismal ritual and not the ritual itself.

Therefore, the teacher, guru, priest, etc. who is "close" to God (enlightened) as it were, is seen as greater than God because he or she can lead the aspirant toward God (knowing who and where God is and how God is to be discovered). Otherwise it would be a very difficult, long and arduous process for the aspirant to realize the truth. It would take millions of incarnations, wherein untold sufferings would occur in the process of gaining experiences which would teach the proper way to discover the Self.

Your journey through this volume will impart one most important point about true spirituality, namely, that true spirituality is universal spirituality. This means that if you discover the truth about your own religion, you will have discovered the truth about all other religions therefore, true religion is a religion of the heart. You must always keep in mind that you are transcendental, immortal and eternal and as such, you are endowed with all the qualities necessary to achieve the highest level of spiritual realization regardless of your background or country of origin.

QUESTION

Why is keeping the company of wise important?

How should a spiritual aspirant think about good association and what actions should they take to insure they will receive and benefit from it?

NOTES:

Another important point is to try to become the best possible disciple you can while still performing your every day duties of life. Once you honestly set in motion the mystical process of your own spiritual aspiration, you will one day encounter more advanced personalities from whom you can learn and progress further in your understanding. In every city, state and country, there exist more advanced personalities who can lead you further along your path of self-discovery. Have you known anyone who is able to control their emotions? Have you known anyone who has lived through a bad situation such as the loss of a loved one or a serious illness and has moved forward with composure, without losing enthusiasm for life? Have you met anyone who has been like a pillar for others, whom others go to in times of trouble or need? If you have the good fortune to know someone like this, get close to them and ask them to show you how they came to possess those advanced spiritual qualities. Ask their permission to spend time with them so that you may benefit from their knowledge and experience in living. You may find that some people are well developed in some areas but not in others. Learn what you can and emulate their virtuous characteristics. If you get to a point where you feel there is no more to learn from that person, continue seeking and you will discover the steps which lead upward on the ladder of spiritual aspiration.

There is no greater blessing than to meet Sages and or Saints who have attained Christ Consciousness, Nirvana, Buddhahood, Heru (Horus)hood, Salvation, Liberation, etc. themselves while at the same time being well versed in the written teachings. They can best help you to understand the subtlety of the teachings and lead you to greater and greater awareness and comprehension which will lead to your own mystical realization in a shorter time than through any other method. They cannot transform you into a spiritual personality; you must do that yourself. However, they can direct you on the correct path and point out your mistakes if you are willing to listen. You need not specifically search for someone who is Enlightened in your own religion.

A disciple who does not practice the teachings of their spiritual preceptor with the notion that the preceptor will provide for his/her spiritual development is like a person who expects to become physically fit by merely going to a gymnasium without doing any exercise. The preceptor provides the mental food in the form of the wisdom teachings and then it is up to you to take this food, consume it, digest it, absorb it and allow it to become part of your being.

Since your innermost self (God) is your Supreme Preceptor, all of the situations you find yourself involved with are divinely inspired to provide for your spiritual education. The same Divine Self is instructing you through the spiritual preceptor and it is this same Divine Self which aids your reflecting and understanding process.

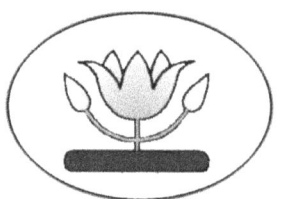

QUESTION

When can you as the aspirant choose those disciplines which suit your personality?

What food does the preceptor provide?

WHO IS A TEACHER

"When the ears of the student are ready to hear, then come the lips of wisdom to fill them with wisdom."

"The lips of the wise are as the doors of a cabinet; no sooner are they opened, but treasures are poured out before you. Like unto trees of gold arranged in beds of silver, are wise sentences uttered in due season."

"The lips of Wisdom are closed, Except to the ears of Understanding."

—Ancient Egyptian Proverbs

When you are growing spiritually you will recognize those who are spiritually advanced. You will be led to them in a mystical way and you will receive the teaching which you need at that time. First you need to begin to purify yourself and make yourself into a good student because only then will you recognize a good teacher. Then you will be fit to receive teachings and to put them into practice because only then will you be ready to understand them.

Spiritual development does not occur in a flash or through a magical touch. It occurs with incremental practice of the teachings as you gradually integrate them into your life through your own self-effort and your level of self-effort determines your level of success. Once you learn the correct methods of spiritual discipline, you can then choose those disciplines (meditation, selfless service, study of scriptures, etc.) which suit your personality and then gradually increase the intensity of your practice even while you carry on the normal duties of life. This process leads to peace and enjoyment of life and to spiritual Enlightenment in an integrated way.

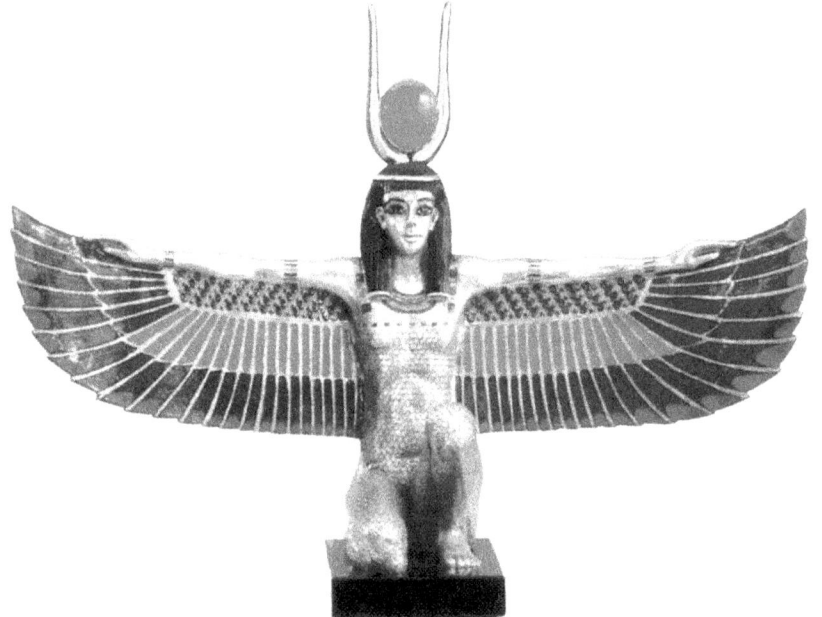

"Rekhat" (Isis – Lady of Wisdom)

Aset (Isis), The Lady of Wisdom, who initiated her son Heru (Horus) into the mysteries of spiritual life and led him to enlightenment and victory against the evil and unrighteousness of Set and his demon associates. She is the supreme wisdom and power behind all priests and priestesses. See **"The Ausarian Resurrection"** by Dr. Muata Abhaya Ashby.

The need for a true teacher of spirituality cannot be overemphasized in the course of spiritual practice. An aspirant is like an athlete. He or she needs coaching and practice in order to attain mastery over the lower self. Every area of your life where you have achieved success, is because you studied and practiced, if not in this lifetime, in a previous

NOTES:

Week 3 Topic: Who is a Teacher?

The need for a true _____ of spirituality cannot be overemphasized in the course of spiritual practice.

one. Spiritual Enlightenment cannot be achieved through magic or through unnatural means. It is achieved through understanding and hard work, not ordinary work, but those activities which lead to purification of the heart.

It is possible to promote your spiritual growth through the books written by genuine spiritual preceptors. The new forms of media such as audio and video have gone even further in conveying the message of the teachings to the entire world. However, at some point, books and tapes can only go so far in explaining the fruits of the true practice of spirituality. This is because the mind can develop many misconceptions and illusions about spirituality just as in any area of ordinary worldly life. Therefore, a guide or coach who is advanced in its practice should be sought out and approached with humility and honesty to ask questions and dispel subtle forms of ignorance. This is the process of spiritual teaching called initiation. The aspirant is initiated into a philosophy and way of life which he or she needs to learn and practice by studying, reflecting and meditating on the teachings. Initiation is a conscious choice to adopt a teaching and to embark on the task of basing your life on it in order to purify your mind and body through the teaching so that you may become a conduit of the divine.

The wisdom texts and scriptures are like a painting of fire. The painting provides an image of what a fire looks like but no warmth emanates from it no matter how close you get. For that, it is necessary to have a real fire. In much the same way, books provide an idea of what is meant by the teachings, however in order to understand their subtlety, something more is needed. A true teacher is one who lives the teaching. Such a one can breathe life into the scriptures and myths to make them understood in the language of today. This is the fire of knowledge which burns away ignorance and illusions which are the cause of human suffering and misery.

There is no nobler occupation than being instructor of Yoga Philosophy, because there is no greater endeavor than relieving the burden of those who are beset by the pain and mental suffering caused by ignorance of their true Self. Also, there is no greater force to dispel the mental anguish of society than Yogic Mystical Philosophy because it gets to the root of psychological complexes in a way that Western psychology does not. Therefore, meeting an authentic teacher of Yoga Philosophy is a highly coveted event by those who have begun to recognize the deeper levels of their own being and the glory of yoga.

One of the main problems of society is the relative lack of interest in the scriptures and secondly, the relatively small number of authentic spiritual preceptors available to teach those who are interested. Many people do not find spirituality attractive because they feel they would "lose" out on life if they became seriously involved. Others see the prospect of spirituality as being too remote for their understanding. They do not realize that their attempts to experience joy from the world are doomed to failure. Further, they do not understand that they already have all they need to be truly happy so they continue to search outside of themselves. These problems arise from the intensification of their ego-body identification and the belief in the erroneous concepts about religion and yoga. Since all souls have emanated from the Higher Self and must some day return to the Self, Yoga is really the ultimate path of all souls. You may choose to procrastinate it however, by being distracted in the phenomenal world of human experiences, but you must realize that you are procrastinating the only true happiness (bliss) which exists in exchange for transient moments of joy followed by pain and suffering. The choice is yours as you are endowed with free will.

An authentic Spiritual Preceptor is not only someone who is advanced on the spiritual path or even just someone who has reached the fully enlightened state. A Guru, in the Upanishadic (teachings of the Indian Upanishads) sense of the word, is someone who is spiritually enlightened and who also is well versed in the scriptural teachings and methods of training aspirants according to their level of understanding. Therefore, a counselor of Yoga must first achieve a high degree of understanding and personal - spiritual emancipation since the subtleties of the mind must be well understood. The teacher must be able to be a refuge for all people, have an extensive knowledge of the teachings pertaining to her/his level of attainment, and enthusiastically pursue all forms of Yoga.

The teaching is often understood differently at different levels. Just as there are different levels of math, such as arithmetic, algebra and calculus, there are different levels of religious practice. The different levels of religion are the Mythological, Ritualistic and the Metaphysical levels. In much the same way, there are varying levels of aspirants who attain to different levels of religious understanding and experience at different times.

QUESTION

(a) A true teacher is one who………………………the teaching

Who is *Sebai*?

Only one who has experienced and matured to greater levels of attainment through *personality integration* can assist others in understanding those higher levels. Here, personality integration refers to the extent that the individual has realized his/her own ego-lessness and identification with the transcendental Self. One on the spiritual path intending to work with and help others, needs to understand the process of initiation and his/her own level of attainment well. Such understanding can only be gained by undergoing the process of practicing the teachings in his/her life. Many teachers (psychologists, psychiatrists, yoga instructors) are deluded as to their understanding of the mind, the philosophy described in the scriptures and of their own attainment. Sometimes, this very delusion causes their failure to cope with the afflictions of others. They are not able to maintain their own peace and serenity and are unable to show others how to deal with their own problems in an effective and lasting way. Therefore, if a teaching is given by one who does not live the teaching or by one who is mistaken about her/his own attainment, that teaching will not be effective.

An authentic teacher of yoga philosophy is someone who is advanced on the path of self-control, one who is indifferent to either positive or negative situations which arise, one who is not affected by praise or censure and is not desirous of any object in the phenomenal world. He or she has discovered inner fulfillment and is a wellspring of joy to all whom they come into contact with. They are not interested in developing relationships with students based on emotionality or other egoistic sensibilities and they are not interested in keeping disciples as servants for their own amusement or in keeping company to inflate their own egos because they have transcended all of these human frailties. They are fulfilled through their realization of their own divinity and help others out of compassion and universal love which flows through them directly from the divine source.

In this manner they help others who seek them out. Acting out the will of the divine which flows through them untouched by egoism, Sages carry out the work of enlightening others. Some aspirants become enlightened in a short time while others in a longer time. The actions of a Sage affect incalculable amounts of people because their actions ripple through the world as a wave ripples across a lake when a stone is thrown into it. By their writings, expositions, their subtle spiritual influence and by their examples as living embodiments of the wisdom, they have an effect on the course of the world and on all whom they come into contact with.

It is acceptable to have advanced yoga students (disciples), provide initial yoga instruction including introduction of exoteric and esoteric knowledge and provide support and encouragement to aspirants, but as a rule, the lower order priests and priestesses does not initiate the disciple into the subtle mysteries of advanced spirituality. This role is reserved for the fully enlightened Guru or spiritual master. A preceptor (*Sebai*) is a spiritual teacher who may or may not have the function of a *guru* or spiritual guide proper. It should be noted here that enlightened personalities are not necessarily nor exclusively to be known as "gurus" although they perform the same function. They may reside in any part of the world and are members of all ethnic groups. Further, they may exist in embodied or non-embodied form. Also, they may be either male or female.

When the *Hem* or priests and priestesses determine that the aspirant is ready to receive the more subtle spiritual instruction of an enlightened personality (*Sebai*), he/she may refer the aspirant for advanced teaching while continuing the counseling-teacher relationship. Therefore, the Upadhyaya and the Guru can complement each other. The Yoga Vasistha emphasizes the importance of teaching the wisdom of the Self as a way of raising one's spiritual consciousness. This is because, by keeping the wisdom of the Self (the Absolute, God) foremost in the mind through the continuous reflectiveness caused by the teaching process, the mind does not stray to sense objects or to other distractions. The mind therefore flows toward the Absolute essential nature, the transcendental Higher Self, at all times.

> In the *Yoga Vasistha,* Sage Vasistha says: One who is ceaselessly devoted to *Brahman**, who exists for the sake of the Self, who rejoices in talking about *Brahman*, and who is engaged in enlightening others about their essential nature, he attains Liberation even in this life. III. 9:1 (*Absolute Self)

In ancient Egypt, the general term for priest or priestess was *Hem or Hemt*. Priesthoods and priestesshoods were also divided into different ranks. There was the *Keri-Eb* or high priest i.e. *Hierophant*. Some of the titles of the Keri-

Question

The actions of a _____ affect incalculable amounts of people

Eb were *"He who sees the secret of heaven"* and *"Chief of the secrets of heaven."* Then came the various levels which handled the administrative duties of the temple which included teaching the mysteries of spirituality as well as the arts, law, writing (hieroglyphics), management, etc. Some of the titles for the various levels of priests were *"The Treasurer of the God"*, *"The scribe of God's House"*, *"The reciter-priest"*, *"The Mete-en-sa"*, *Scribe of the altar"* and *Superintendent of the House of God."* Judges were also part of the priesthood. They specifically belonged to the following of Goddess *MAAT*. The largest priesthoods belonged to the Temples of the Gods Amun, Asar, Ra and Heru, and the Goddesses *Net, Aset* and *Hetheru.* These Goddesses are also known by other names which are given according to the mystical symbolism of the teachings. These include Isis, Nephthys, Bast, Mut, Nekhebet, Uatchet, and all other forms of the Goddess.[2]

A reference to the ancient Egyptian view concerning a *Hierophant* or teacher of the mysteries comes from *Philo of Alexandria*. Philo was a mystic practitioner of the Egyptian mysteries and Gnostic Christianity. Gnostic Christianity is an outgrowth of ancient Egyptian Religion. Gnosticism includes mystical writings in Coptic and Greek language about the nature of the soul and of creation along with mystical wisdom and philosophy which lead to mystical awareness. Orthodox Christianity or the Roman and Byzantine Catholicism which survives to this day originated out of Christian Gnosticism.

In reference to the "Divine Spirit" and "Moses", Philo gives the following instruction:

> "It [the Divine Spirit] is [ever] present with only one class of men—with those who, having stripped themselves of all things in genesis, even to the innermost veil and garment of opinion, come unto God with minds unclothed and naked."
>
> "And so Moses, having fixed his tent outside the camp—that is, the whole of the body—that is to say, having made firm his mind, so that it does not move, begins to worship God and entering into the most holy mysteries. And he becomes, not only a *mystes*, but also a Hierophant of revelations, and teacher of divine things, which he will indicate to those who have had their ears made pure. With such kind of men the Divine Spirit is ever present, guiding their every way aright."

Philo directly addresses the idea of divine inspiration using Moses, whom the Bible states was an Egyptian Priest, as an example. Philo's description of the "meeting" between God and Moses is an example of the orthodox versus the Gnostic understanding and practice of spirituality. While the orthodox view presents this meeting as Moses being conscious of himself as a person looking at God who is outside of himself, the Gnostic understanding is that God is communed with, by setting aside the ego consciousness. Further on, Philo states that it is when this ecstasy occurs (*having fixed his tent outside the camp*) that the true worship of God begins. It is this ecstasy which provides real insight into one's own spiritual nature and which bestows the highest ability to teach others about the mysteries of the soul.

This point is very important for a serious aspirant to understand. As a worshipper of the Divine, if you maintain yourself separate within your mind and body and hold onto your ego, you are only practicing a ritualistic form of worship. This form of superficial practice of spirituality will not bestow true knowledge on you. Rather, your knowledge will be based on the information you are able to gather from your mind and senses which are limited and conditioned.

> *"Strive to see with the inner eye, the heart. It sees the reality not subject to emotional or personal error; it sees the essence. Intuition then is the most important quality to develop."*
> —Ancient Egyptian Proverb

In most orthodox (adhering to traditional or established beliefs) forms of religion, the worshiper is mentally aware of him/herself as being an individual looking at another individual (God) in the form of pictures, idols, scriptural

---

[2] for more detailes on the levels of the Ancient Egyptian clergy see the book *Egyptian Mysteries* by Dr. Muata Ashby

Question

Where was the largest priesthood?

NOTES:

descriptions, etc. In Gnostic or mystical forms of religion (Egyptian mysteries, Vedanta, Taoism, Buddhism, Gnostic Christianity) which employ yoga philosophy and meditation techniques, the worshiper is directed to cease the thoughts of the mind which involve personal identification with the body and ego and thereby become one with the Absolute by an immediate, direct, intuitive knowledge of God, the ultimate reality. This intuitive knowledge refers to a personal religious experience in Gnosticism. A contrast should be drawn here between the mystical-ecstatic experience (just defined) and the ritualistic religious experience. The ritualistic or surface level religious experience is often accompanied by heightened emotions, visions and other phenomena, however there is no transcendental vision of the Absolute and no transcendence of the ego-self. In other words, an ecstatic religious experience at the level of the mind and senses does not show you that you are not the body, mind and senses and does not reveal your true Self.

Lastly, it would be an exceedingly great error for someone to claim to be a realized spiritual master if they are not. This is because the psychic illusion that would be created within their own mind would hamper their own spiritual movement. However, the imitation of spiritual personalities and their behavior is permitted and even promoted to the extent that it is grounded in reality and honesty. The idea is that we are what we feel, act, believe and think. Therefore, as we feel, act, believe and think in a particular way, we become like onto that. Thus, it is all right to emulate the qualities of a Sage because this process helps to control the ego and develop sagely qualities. Generally, self-realized masters do not go around proclaiming their enlightenment. Rather, it is more the case that their disciples are drawn to them because of their teachings and example. The advancing aspirant can know who is an advanced personality due to his/her own increasing purity and wisdom. Therefore, in order to recognize a true teacher, you need to develop your own intuitive faculties. This is accomplished by studying the teachings and by developing serenity and strong moral character.

The Role of the Teacher

The teacher does not become sentimentally involved with students, feel sorrow for those who do not follow the teachings or elation over those who do. The teacher, having discovered the source of pain and suffering, seeks to eliminate it wherever it may be, through the force of wisdom which, like the Eye of Ra, burns away all ignorance in its path. Where there is wisdom there can be no ignorance and therefore, no pain and suffering, just as there can be no darkness in a room where the light has been turned on. However, the teacher does not seek to violate anyone's freedom of will. Those who wish to be under the guiding influence of the teacher must do so out of free will, since not even a teacher of the highest power can remove their pain and ignorance if they do not want to become enlightened. Therefore, a teacher makes him or herself a conduit, an instrument for the Divine through which the Divine may enlighten others when they are ready. In the mean time, nature (Neters) through the unseen mysterious force of Meskhenet (karma) guides souls who are not ready to receive the teaching of the advanced Spiritual Preceptor. The path of nature is the path of spiritual growth through many life times and requires the experience of many sorrows, disappointments, disillusionments and violence. However, these events are planned by nature to awaken the deeper need of the soul to seek spiritual enlightenment through wisdom rather than through the world of sense enjoyments and complicated karmic entanglements.

The teacher, by becoming an example and transcending the pain and sorrow of human existence, can then express true compassion for humanity. So the most effective way to help humanity is to help yourself to become enlightened. Then the obstacles which trouble most people will not affect you in the least. Your wisdom and realization will be as an armor which protects you against the miseries of the world. Even the most sincere social workers cannot help humanity to the fullest if they themselves are suffering from the maladies of human existence. If you do not know how to swim in the ocean of the world of human experiences, you cannot save others from drowning. The large number of psychologists and psychiatrists who experience problems such as stress and commit suicide is an example of this. Therefore, unless you are above being affected by the human condition by working to overcome it in yourself through yogic science, you cannot assist those who are affected by that condition.

NOTES:

Topic" The role of a Teacher?

The teacher makes him or herself………………….. and……………………………..for the Divine through which the…………………..

While there is always a value to any action an ordinary person takes to uplift society (value to society and to themselves), the most effective way to change the world is to begin changing yourself. As Jesus said: *seek ye first the kingdom of Heaven, and his righteousness; and all these things shall be added to you.* While continuing to work for the betterment of humanity, you must not take on the burdens of the world upon your shoulders. You must trust and have faith in the plan of NETER (God) who works through the Neters (the Neters-mysterious divine forces of nature and the cosmos). You must honestly understand that your own need to help society and rectify injustice is an expression of your own need to achieve wholeness and this wholeness cannot be found in the world from an egoistic perspective. If you do not trust in nature's ability to help others, it is like saying that you do not trust in God, that God's creation (the world) is imperfect and unjust. This would be an expression of your own ignorance.

> *"Salvation is accomplished through the efforts of the individual. There is no mediator between man and his / her salvation."*
>
> —Ancient Egyptian Proverb

You cannot assist others who do not want to be assisted or who are not qualified to receive the teachings of mystical spirituality (Yoga philosophy). You can only work to purify your heart and to promote the same in others by your example and be prepared for the time when they will seek your assistance. This does not mean that you cannot or should not engage in projects to help others. To the contrary, such projects can help you to develop purity of heart by providing experiences and opportunities for you to practice selflessness, self-control, dispassion, detachment, etc. and thereby promote effacement of the ego. The key is in the attitude with which you perform your duties. If you engage in actions with an attitude of egoistic attachment, pride, selfishness, repulsion or regret, you will intensify the fetters which bind you to human existence. This attitude would be like rejecting God's plan for your spiritual development. If you treat all of your experiences as opportunities to do divine work by allowing your soul to express itself through your mind and body when serving others and developing the latent talents within you, then your experiences will lead to inner fulfillment and mental serenity which will open the path of self-discovery. This is the true purpose of social work.

Every day, Nature (God) provides you with opportunities to purify your heart. All situations in life are carefully planned tests for you to practice developing divine virtues: humility, selflessness, detachment, positive state of mind, fearlessness, joy, etc. The teachings of Maat show you how to achieve these goals through your actions in daily activities. In reality, you enter the Hall of Maat to be judged every day of your life. The world of human experiences is the Hall of Maat. From a higher perspective, this entire universe is the Hall of Maat.

> *"GOD is truth (Maat), and GOD has established the earth thereupon."*
>
> —Ancient Egyptian Proverb

Therefore, you should strive to understand the way of *Maat* in order to come into harmony with the way of the universe. When you consciously commence this process, you will begin to discover the true joy of life and those around you will benefit in a most profound and mysterious way, perhaps even without your knowing it. If you allow yourself to be guided by the teachings of wisdom, you will be entering the stream of light which flows from the Divine, from the highest to the lowest. Having done this you will have enlisted the help of the greatest power that exists, your own Higher Self. Then, wherever you go and whatever you do will be blessed with the Divine essence. This is the way of Maat which puts the forces of nature at your command to do divine work. When you consciously decide to align yourself with the forces of wisdom as opposed to the forces of ignorance and egoism by changing your life through the ancient practices of mystical spirituality, you have initiated yourself on the path to enlightenment and salvation. Thus, initiation is a deeply personal and serious matter which you need to reflect upon. True transformation can occur only if you are sincere and honest with yourself and if you follow the practices as instructed. Therefore, spiritual life is not easy in the beginning but it is most rewarding in the end. It confers the greatest goal of life, eternal bliss which is not perishable like worldly attainments.

Question

The key is in the _____ attitude with which you perform your duties

How to Approach a Spiritual Preceptor

There are many orders of priests and priestesses but the Seba is the imparter of mysteries to the initiates. This is a special personality, someone who has achieved Divine Consciousness, which is the goal of all spiritual efforts. Those personalities have chosen to maintain the initiatic tradition and instruct new aspirants who will become initiates and eventually priests and priestesses as well as Preceptors. Gaining an insight into who they are and how to approach them is of paramount importance in achieving the higher goals of spiritual development. You may begin by reading the books of those personalities so as to have a partial communion with their minds and then you will want to meet them in person in order to truly understand what you have read!

There are many people who do their own research and believe they have discovered the "mysteries" and thus they go around teaching others and sometimes even starting new religions but in the end their lack of authenticity emerges in the form of egoism, unrighteousness, inability to handle crisis, inability to resist worldly temptations, inability to show others the path to spiritual realization beyond slogans, exuberant rantings or emotional appeals. Many preachers use exciting methods to talk about their scriptures and may even sound authentic but the excitement soon dies down and the aspirant is left without a viable understanding or path to follow. Also, many self-styled spiritual leaders are not interested in showing others a higher path because then they would loose their source of income. An authentic Spiritual Preceptor is not interested in developing cults, slaves, servants or keeping people at an ignorant level.

An authentic teacher is and should be treated as a precious resource, even more so than millions of dollars in the bank. Why? Because that person will free you from untold mysteries over many future lifetimes and they will lead you to enlightenment in this lifetime so that you can truly enjoy whatever wealth you have. Even if you are poor you will also be led to enjoyment of life since the successful aspirants transcend all good or bad conditions in the world.

You should approach the preceptor with humility and not insolently. As soon as the authentic teacher hears arrogance, conceit, self-importance, vanity, snobbishness, etc., their lips close and the flow if the enlightening stream of the river to enlightenment ceases to flow towards you. Even if you egoistically sought to attend their class you would not understand or benefit from the teaching. Respect, humility deference and obedience are keys to approaching a preceptor. Without these your relationship cannot exist. For this reason you should practice Maat and get rid of the gross (overt) impurities (anger, hatred, greed, jealousy, lust, envy, etc.) in your personality. The preceptor will show you how to get rid of the more subtle (unconscious) impurities so that you may progress in the teaching.

> (4)"Have faith in your master's ability to lead you along the path of truth"
>
> -Ancient Egyptian precept for the initiates.

Also, never take the preceptor for granted. Never treat or refer to the preceptor as you would a "friend" or a "buddy" or as "one of the guys." Also, as the preceptor is elevated in consciousness but operating through a physical body, there will possibly be human occasional error or faults in areas outside of the teachings. An ignorant aspirant would look at this with the idea that enlightenment means absolute perfection in everything and in this manner dismiss the teacher as inadequate and thus loose out on the benefits that would otherwise be derived from the association. Therefore, as in ordinary relations, there should never be gossiping about faults or petty foibles or minor eccentricities.

> *"It takes a strong disciple to rule over the mountainous thoughts and constantly go to the essence of the meaning; as mental complexity increases, thus will the depth of your decadence and challenge both be revealed."*
>
> -Ancient Egyptian Proverb

Ordinary friendships, based on egoism, are burdened with egoistic desires and expectations. A preceptor is not interested in fulfilling your egoistic desires but rather in dispelling these. Therefore, if you do not have the

Question

Many preachers use _____ methods?

understanding as to what is the nature and purpose of the initiatic affiliation your relationship on that basis is doomed and you will be the one leaving the relationship without transforming, without growing and enlightening yourself. Never treat the preceptor as an ordinary person who like others has an "opinion" you can accept or disregard. If you want to be a "free spirit," to exercise "free will" you have no need of the preceptor. If you are a sincere aspirant you will have no need to exercise free will to commit sinful acts or unrighteous schemes, nor will you need to reserve the right to hurt others or delude yourself. Therefore, your free will can be surrendered to the Divine without a second thought or reservation. Once you are secure in the authenticity of the person you have chosen as your teacher you must realize that that person is a representative of the Divine on earth and should be accorded the same respect and admiration as a facilitator who will help you on the path. You have come to that person because you recognize your ignorance and the elevation of the teacher. Therefore, cease all thoughts of pride and self-importance. Otherwise you are only toying at being an aspirant and have no chance to be a real initiate. As you check out a teacher yes you should be cautious and slow to ally yourself, but once you choose to do so your allegiance should be complete and unreserved, unconditional and wholehearted. The unrighteous and therefore, limited ways of relating thwart the spiritual process of the teacher disciple relationship and will render it fruitless. They cause rifts in the mind of the aspirant and prevent them from pursuing the teaching in the correct manner. Sometimes as children, they may keep themselves from facing the preceptor after they have made some transgression, due to pride and shame. At these times when life humbles the aspirant it is even more important that they should trust in the teacher who will never rub their noses in it or turn them away. A preceptor is like the sun, who witnesses the good and the bad but yet remains aloof, dispassionate but yet in touch. So the preceptor understands how tough it is to make it through the gross and subtle temptations, fancies, notions and desires of life and is thus prepared to forgive all. Even though a transcendent master is beyond personal hang-ups, desires, attachments and so on an aspirant should never disrespect the preceptor, steal from the preceptor (objects or knowledge) or speak out of turn or test the patience of the preceptor. Some aspirants, due to ignorance, believe they can go around taking knowledge from different teachers without giving anything in return. So they remain unchanged because they do not give themselves, their allegiance, trust and support to the cause of the teacher. Therefore, they never get the opportunity to form a long-term relationship with the teacher which they need in order to develop deeper understanding of the teaching. Their understanding remains superficial and thereby they develop delusions of grandeur as advanced initiates and in reality they are setting themselves up for a great fall.

> *"Sacrifice the first portions of the harvest, that your strength and faith to bring about what you desire may be increased; give the FIRST portion, to avoid danger of worldly indulgence; Give that you may receive. Fulfill the requirements of the universal law of equilibrium"*
>
> -Ancient Egyptian Proverb

Every aspirant must offer their ego, pride and ignorance on the divine altar of wisdom. They must sacrifice the egoistic notions, and vanity in order to attain insight and wisdom. They must pledge their service to the preceptor in the form of physical, mental and spiritual support and devotion. Further, an aspirant should not hesitate to beg the preceptor's forgiveness for any transgression. While the preceptor is not personally bothered by transgressions or insolence, etc. the preceptor's voice is silenced in the presence of such ignorant aspirants and this hurts them severely, allowing the cycle of ignorance pain and suffering in life and reincarnation to continue unabated. Disrespect and callousness as well as ill manners and rudeness are symptoms of spiritual immaturity, i.e. ignorance. Spiritual teachings to such a personality will be as effective as a instructing a dog or a cat on the finer principles of brain surgery. This unrighteous way of relating closes the door to real spiritual instruction. And this closing has been the fault of the aspirant. Take care to not be two faced and burn your bridges, thinking that you have attained some higher level and no longer need your teacher or discovered a better teacher, and thus disrespecting the old. The old brought you to the new you think you have arrived at and is therefore worthy of the same respect and gratitude that was supposed to have been there all along. While the teacher exists in transcendental bliss regardless of the aspirant's righteous conduct or lack thereof the aspirant is severely affected by their actions. Even the subtlest unrighteous act is a pathway to strengthening of the ego and egoism leads to impaired intellect and degraded feeling. Unrighteous behavior reverberates in the consciousness of an aspirant and forms negative impressions in the mind that clout understanding and may take lifetimes to erase. Therefore, take care to make sure that your relationship with the preceptor is righteous if not in the beginning, certainly in the end. But there is only one true ending if it can be referred to as such and that is the attainment of enlightenment. Does a river end when it joins the ocean? In like manner the

Question:

When life humbles the aspirant it is even more important that they should do what?

How should a spiritual aspirant think and feel about humbling themselves to the teaching and their teacher?

true end of the road of the teacher disciple relationship is the aspirants attainment of enlightenment but this is not the end but a merging of the aspirants consciousness with that of the teacher, the beginning of conscious experience of the transcendental spirit and here begins also the journey of the aspirant who has now become a preceptor and this is the initiatic tradition, which reaches back to the far reaches of time all the way back to the first aspirants, those who learned from God (Djehuty) directly and became preceptors to those who followed next and so on up to the present.

You must treat a Spiritual Preceptor even better than you treat someone you love. Ordinary love affairs are fraught with strife, love and hate periods sprinkled with passionate moments and dashes of exuberant flights of fancy. People develop possessiveness and attachments and call these love and also they fall in out of love as if it were a disease. This of course is not true love. True love transcends even the capacity to feel anger or disdain. If you truly love something you stick with it through thick or thin and there is no "falling out" of it. It is an upward and expanding movement that is all encompassing and eternal. So unless you have loved in this way do not believed that you have truly loved for loved anything. Your relationships are only training you for the true love and you must learn that from the preceptor.[3]

You must attempt to never lose your temper in the presence of the preceptor and never treat the preceptor unrighteously or with resentment. You must learn to receive whatever the teacher says and apply it in your life. Many aspirants have learned to do things "their own way" instead of following instructions from the teacher. You may question for deeper understanding but not to challenge in order to get out of your duty or to discredit what has been said so that you may feel justified in disobeying the edict. That is the path of the weak minded and the ignorant. Never attempt to put emotional guilt trips on elevated personalities. These are immature attempts and getting the desires of your ego and they will be impotent in the face of the elevated preceptor. Gossiping about the preceptor or any other person is also a sign of degraded consciousness and will eventually lead you away from the teacher as well as true spiritual knowledge. Bouncing around from one teacher to another is also a way to go astray, as you cannot find water if you dig several superficial wells, but rather a single deep well. Therefore, even though you may read the books of many teachers or see many teachers there should be one special one with whom you may develop a rapport that will cause the flow of divine wisdom to move in your direction. Therefore, seek out a teacher who has a personality that is in harmony with your own. That is, if you are an intellectual person, look for a teacher who emphasizes the wisdom aspect of the disciplines. However, while you may have a special resonance in some aspect of the teachings there should always be practice of the other disciplines so that you may develop your entire personality and not be like the fanatical ignorant masses. Also, you must strive to never say you will do something for the teacher and then not do it or develop excuses. All of these things and more are for the world and will not bring you the favor of the preceptor. Favor is attention and when you have this the lips of the preceptor move for you as they will not for others and you will receive the grace of insight into Divine Consciousness that is the objective of all aspirants the world over.

Aspirants should take care to pay their dues. This means that at no time should they allow themselves to believe that they have achieved anything on their own or without the assistance of mentors and teachers. There are many unrighteous writers who take the writings of others and give no credit to them and even act as if they themselves wrote the information. In like manner some aspirants conduct discourses on the teachings and do not give the proper credit for what they have learned and thereby develop egoism as they dazzle others with their "wisdom." However, as they fatten their own ego they are actually leading people to a place that they will not be able to lead them beyond and here is where stagnation in the teachings commences. Some preachers rely on drama or exuberant performances while giving sermons. This distracts people and may even make people believe that these preachers or lecturers know what they are talking about but the listeners will not be able to transform themselves because the teaching is dishonest and incomplete. If an aspirant does not pay homage to the teacher they are committing an injustice and the higher wisdom will escape them even if it be presented to them or even if they come across it in a book.

Approach with a spirit of service and do not practice the mysteries as a part-time dabler. In order to progress you must work diligently and learn how every waking moment is to be dedicated to the Divine. This is the only way to succeed in dispelling the veil of ignorance. The world is a very powerful force with the ignorant mind and an

---

[3] See the book *Egyptian Tantra Yoga*

Question

You must attempt to never lose your_____

aspirant must fight hard to overcome the yoke of worldly consciousness. Only complete dedication and service towards the Divine will open the doors of the House of Asar (palace of enlightenment). Therefore, you must understand that being an initiate means complete devotion to spiritual life and this translates to reverence and service towards the Spiritual Preceptor. Never allow the preceptor to do work that you can do since their time should be reserved for the higher dissemination of the teachings. So again, in serving the teacher you are facilitating the teachers time and availability to teach you and others. The teacher may not always ask for help because he/she wants to give you room to act on initiative. Thereby the initiatic process cannot be one-sided. The aspirant who hopes to become an *initiate* needs to *initiate* the contact with the teacher and have the *initiative* to make good use of the teaching.

You may find a Spiritual Preceptor who has all the qualifications to lead you, someone who is not only elevated but also who is capable of teaching you how to elevate yourself, for the two capacities are not the same nor are they always found in the same personality. A person may be elevated but not versed in the scripture or the ways to develop aspirants. Therefore, if you feel a burning desire to grow spiritually and you have dealt with your worldly responsibilities so that you can be free to pursue the teaching seek out a teacher. That person may be in your hometown but if not you must go to them and touch the floor with your face before them and humbly ask for their permission to be accepted as a student. First though, develop a keen understanding of what it means to be an aspirant and become familiar with and practice the disciplines of Maat which purify the heart. Do not present to God a dirty vessel. Wouldn't you wash a bow before placing food in it as an offering to God? In the same manner, your presentation of your personality before a preceptor as if to God herself. Therefore, be clean in your body, mind and soul to the best of your ability, then, even if you have to go around the world to meet and work with your teacher the trip will not be a waste of time but a glorious start on the golden road to enlightened experience.

The Concept of Sebai

The Sebai in Ancient Egypt

<u>The Term Sebai means "Illuminer of the mysteries"</u>

The highest company an aspirant can keep is with the Sabai. In Ancient Egypt the priests and priestesses were revered as enlightened councilors and spiritual leaders or sages who lead initiates to meet the Divine. There are few cases where they are canonized or considered as gods and goddesses as such. Imhotep is one such example. However, in their capacity they were charged with becoming one with the divinities during rituals in order to bring forth the glory of that divinity. Thus, in Kamitan spirituality there is more focus on the divinity as opposed to the personality of the preceptor as concerns reverence in the form of an incarnate divinity. That form of reverence and devotion was reserved for the Per-Aah or phearoah. The priests and priestesses were facilitators and enlightened guides to the mysteries. As enlightened personalities they were hailed as leaders and directors of of society.

The kind of reverence towards priests and priestesses that developed in India was unknown in Ancient Egypt. Rather, the mysteries were kept closely amongst the initiates within the temple system and the public was only allowed to participate in the holidays, traditions and public festivals. The teaching was disseminated within the temple system and it was god and the teaching which were the primary focus and not the spiritual preceptor. It was perhaps, in their wisdom that the Kemetic priests and priestesses sought to avoid the situation which has developed in modern India, that the teachings are so proliferated that there are many charlatans throughout the country, conning the common folk.

Question

In Kamitan spirituality there is more focus on the _____ as opposed to the personality of the _____.

The Fundamental Principles of Neterian Religion

NETERIANISM
(The Oldest Known Religion in History)

The term "Neterianism" is derived from the name "Shetaut Neter." Shetaut Neter means the "Hidden Divinity." It is the ancient philosophy and mythic spiritual culture that gave rise to the Ancient Egyptian civilization. Those who follow the spiritual path of Shetaut Neter are therefore referred to as "Neterians." The fundamental principles common to all denominations of Neterian Religion may be summed up as follows.

What is Neterianism and Who are the Neterians?

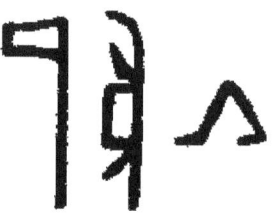

"Shemsu Neter"

"Follower (of) Neter"

The term "Neterianism" is derived from the name "Shetaut Neter." Those who follow the spiritual path of Shetaut Neter are therefore referred to as "Neterians."

Neterianism is the science of Neter, that is, the study of the secret or mystery of Neter, the enigma of that which transcends ordinary consciousness but from which all creation arises. The world did not come from nothing, nor is it sustained by nothing. Rather it is a manifestation of that which is beyond time and space but which at the same time permeates and maintains the fundamental elements. In other words, it is the substratum of Creation and the essential nature of all that exists.

So those who follow the Neter may be referred to as Neterians.

NOTES:

The world did not come from _____.

Where did the term "Neterianism" derive from?

_____

Those who follow the path may be referred to as _____

Neterian Great Truths

1. **"Pa Neter ua ua Neberdjer m Neteru"** -"The Neter, the Supreme Being, is One and alone and as Neberdjer, manifesting everywhere and in all things in the form of Gods and Goddesses."

Neberdjer means "all-encompassing divinity," the all-inclusive, all-embracing Spirit which pervades all and who is the ultimate essence of all. This first truth unifies all the expressions of Kamitan religion.

2. **"an-Maat swy Saui Set s-Khemn"** - "Lack of righteousness brings fetters to the personality and these fetters lead to ignorance of the Divine."

When a human being acts in ways that contradict the natural order of nature, negative qualities of the mind will develop within that person's personality. These are the afflictions of Set. Set is the neteru of egoism and selfishness. The afflictions of Set include: anger, hatred, greed, lust, jealousy, envy, gluttony, dishonesty, hypocrisy, etc. So to be free from the fetters of set one must be free from the afflictions of Set.

3. **"s-Uashu s-Nafu n saiu Set"** -"Devotion to the Divine leads to freedom from the fetters of Set."

To be liberated (Nafu - freedom - to breath) from the afflictions of Set, one must be devoted to the Divine. Being devoted to the Divine means living by Maat. Maat is a way of life that is purifying to the heart and beneficial for society as it promotes virtue and order. Living by Maat means practicing Shedy (spiritual practices and disciplines).

Uashu means devotion and the classic pose of adoring the Divine is called "Dua," standing or sitting with upraised hands facing outwards towards the image of the divinity.

4. **"ari Shedy Rekh ab m Maakheru"** - "The practice of the Shedy disciplines leads to knowing oneself and the Divine. This is called being True of Speech."

Doing Shedy means to study profoundly, to penetrate the mysteries (Shetaut) and discover the nature of the Divine.

There have been several practices designed by the sages of Ancient Kamit to facilitate the process of self-knowledge.

These are the religious (Shetaut) traditions and the Sema (Smai) Tawi (yogic) disciplines related to them that augment the spiritual practices.

All the traditions relate the teachings of the sages by means of myths related to particular gods or goddesses. It is understood that all of these neteru are related, like brothers and sisters, having all emanated from the same source, the same Supremely Divine parent, who is neither male nor female, but encompasses the totality of the two.

NOTES:

Write out the Four Great Truths.

What are the afflictions of Set?

What is the meaning of the term "Nafu"?

The Great Truths of Neterianism are realized by means of Four Spiritual Disciplines in Three Steps

The four disciples are: Rekh Shedy (Wisdom), Ari Shedy (Righteous Action and Selfless Service), Uashu (Ushet) Shedy (Devotion) and Uaa Shedy (Meditation)

The Three Steps are: Listening, Ritual, and Meditation

SEDJM REKH SHEDY

LISTEN

- **Sedjm REKH Shedy** - **Listening** to the WISDOM of the Neterian Traditions

    - Shetaut Asar — Teachings of the Asarian Tradition
    - Shetaut Anu — Teachings of the Ra Tradition
    - Shetaut Menefer — Teachings of the Ptah Tradition
    - Shetaut Waset — Teachings of the Amun Tradition
    - Shetaut Netrit — Teachings of the Goddess Tradition
    - Shetaut Aton — Teachings of the Aton Tradition

ARI SHEDY

RITUAL

- **Ari Maat Shedy** – **Righteous Actions** – Purifies the GROSS impurities of the Heart

    - Maat Shedy — True Study of the Ways of hidden nature of Neter
    - Maat Aakhu — True Deeds that lead to glory
    - Maat Aru — True Ritual

UASHU (USHET) SHEDY

- **Ushet Shedy** – **Devotion to the Divine** – Purifies the EMOTIONAL impurities of the Heart

    - Shmai — Divine Music
    - Sema Paut — Meditation in motion
    - Neter Arit — Divine Offerings – Selfless-Service – virtue -

UAA SHEDY

MEDITATE

- **Uaa m Neter Shedy** - 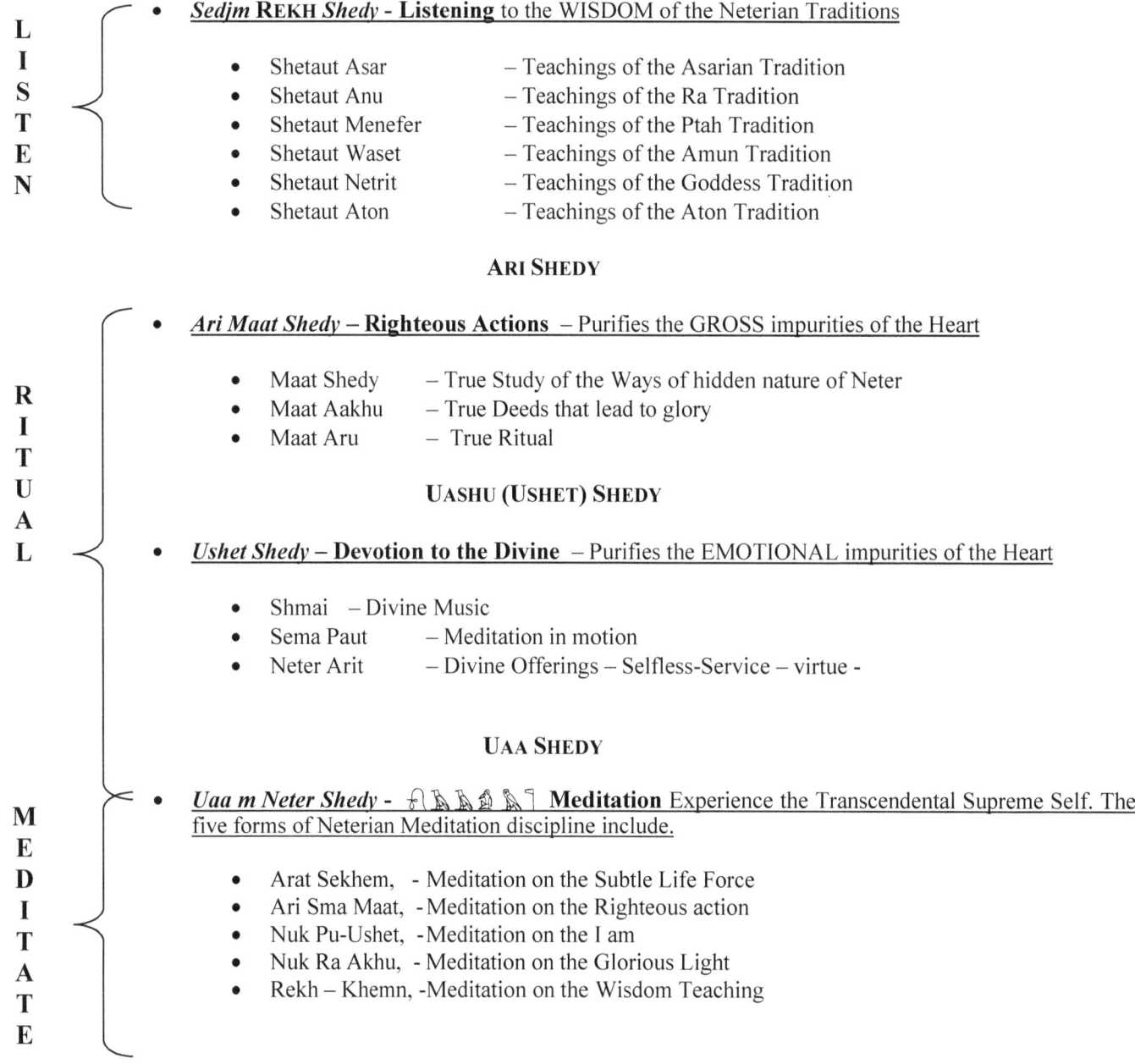 **Meditation** Experience the Transcendental Supreme Self. The five forms of Neterian Meditation discipline include.

    - Arat Sekhem, - Meditation on the Subtle Life Force
    - Ari Sma Maat, - Meditation on the Righteous action
    - Nuk Pu-Ushet, - Meditation on the I am
    - Nuk Ra Akhu, - Meditation on the Glorious Light
    - Rekh – Khemn, - Meditation on the Wisdom Teaching

NOTES:

The four disciplines of Shedy are:

_____

_____

_____

_____

Summary of The Great Truths and the Shedy Paths to their Realization

Great Truths

Shedy Disciplines

I

God is One and in all things manifesting through the Neteru

I

Listen to the Wisdom Teachings (Become Wise)
Learn the mysteries as taught by an authentic teacher which allows this profound statement to be understood.

II

Unrighteousness brings fetters and these cause ignorance of truth

(#1)

II

Acting (Living) by Truth
Apply the Philosophy of right action to become virtuous and purify the heart

III

Devotion to God allows the personality to free itself from the fetters

III

Devotion to the Divine
Worship, ritual and divine love allows the personality purified by truth to eradicate the subtle ignorance that binds it to mortal existence.

IIII

The Shedy disciplines are the greatest form of worship of the Divine

IIII

Meditation
Allows the whole person to go beyond the world of time and space and the gross and subtle ignorance of mortal human existence to discover that which transcends time and space.

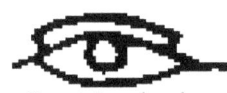

Great Awakening
Occurs when all of the Great Truths have been realized by perfection of the Shedy disciplines to realize their true nature and actually experience oneness with the transcendental Supreme Being.

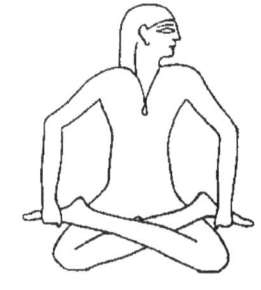

Question

Great _____ occurs when all of the Great Truths have been realized.

The Neterian Creed

As a *Neterian*, I follow the Ancient African-Kamitan religious path of *Shetaut Neter*, which teaches about the mysteries of the Supreme Being, <u>*Neberdjer*</u>, the All Encompassing Divinity. I believe that from *Neberdjer* proceed all the *Neteru* (gods and goddesses), and all the worlds, and the entire universe. Since *Neberdjer* manifests as the *Neteru*, *Neberdjer* can be worshipped as a god or a goddess. I believe that there is only one Supreme Being, *Neberdjer*, and that the gods and goddesses are expressions of the One Supreme Being, *Neberdjer*. As a Neterian, I strive to come into harmony with the gods and goddesses, the *Neteru*, by developing within my personality the different virtuous and divine qualities they symbolize; this will lead me closer to *Neberdjer*. As a Neterian, I also believe that Supreme Being I call *Neberdjer* is the same Supreme Being that is worshiped by other religions under different names.

I believe that *Neberdjer* established all creation on *Maat*, righteousness, truth, and order, and that my actions, termed *Ari*, determine the quality of life I lead and experience. If I act with *Maat* (positive *Ari*) my path will be free of suffering and pain. When I forget *Maat* and act in an unrighteous manner (negative *Ari*), I invite suffering and pain into my life.

As a *Neterian* I believe when my body dies, my heart's actions will be examined against *Maat*. If it is found that I upheld *Maat* during my lifetime, I will have positive *Ari*, and my *Akhu* (spirit) will become one with *Neberdjer* for all eternity. This is called *Nehast*, the Spiritual Awakening-Enlightenment. If it is found that I acted with selfishness and greed, I will have negative *Ari*, and my *Ba* (soul) will suffer after death and then be reincarnated again to live in the world of time and space again. This is called *Uhemankh* (reincarnation).

As a *Neterian* I believe in the teaching of *Shemsu*, following the path of *Shetaut Neter*, by practicing the disciplines of *Shedy*, which include: Study of Wisdom teachings (*Rech-Ab*), Devotion to God (*Uashu*), Acting with Righteousness (*Maat*) and Meditation (*Uaa*). *Neberdjer* provided the *Shetitu*, the spiritual teaching that was written in *Medu Neter* (hieroglyphic scripture) so that the *Shemsu* (followers) might study the wisdom teaching of Shetaut Neter. Two most important *Neterian* scriptures are the *Pert M Hru* and the *Hessu Amun*, and the most important *Neterian* myth is the *Asarian* Resurrection.

By the practice of the disciplines of Shedy, I will discover the *Shetaut* (Mysteries) of life and become *Maakheru*, Pure of Heart. I will become one with God even before death, and I will discover supreme peace, abiding happiness and fulfillment of my life's purpose, and promote peace and harmony for the world.

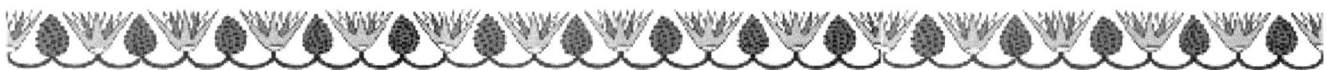

Question

What teaching(s) of the Neterian Creed do you believe in currently, are working on believing, find hard to believe? Why?

How should a spiritual aspirant think about the prospect of "becoming godlike" and their capacity to live a life of virtue and cultivation of the spirit through scientific knowledge, practice and bodily discipline and is this possible for everyone? If so why so? If not why not?

The Spiritual Culture and the Purpose of Life: Shetaut Neter

> "Men and women are to become God-like through a life of virtue and the cultivation of the spirit through scientific knowledge, practice and bodily discipline."
>
> -Ancient Egyptian Proverb

The highest forms of Joy, Peace and Contentment are obtained when the meaning of life is discovered. When the human being is in harmony with life, then it is possible to reflect and meditate upon the human condition and realize the limitations of worldly pursuits. When there is peace and harmony in life, a human being can practice any of the varied disciplines designated as Shetaut Neter to promote {his/her} evolution towards the ultimate goal of life, which Spiritual Enlightenment. Spiritual Enlightenment is the awakening of a human being to the awareness of the Transcendental essence which binds the universe and which is eternal and immutable. In this discovery is also the sobering and ecstatic realization that the human being is one with that Transcendental essence. With this realization comes great joy, peace and power to experience the fullness of life and to realize the purpose of life during the time on earth. The lotus is a symbol of Shetaut Neter, meaning the turning towards the light of truth, peace and transcendental harmony.

Shetaut Neter

We have established that the Ancient Egyptians were African peoples who lived in the north-eastern quadrant of the continent of Africa. They were descendants of the Nubians, who had themselves originated from farther south into the heart of Africa at the Great Lakes region, the sources of the Nile River. They created a vast civilization and culture earlier than any other society in known history and organized a nation that was based on the concepts of balance and order as well as spiritual enlightenment. These ancient African people called their land Kamit, and soon after developing a well-ordered society, they began to realize that the world is full of wonders, but also that life is fleeting, and that there must be something more to human existence. They developed spiritual systems that were designed to allow human beings to understand the nature of this secret being who is the essence of all Creation. They called this spiritual system "Shtaut Ntr (Shetaut Neter)."

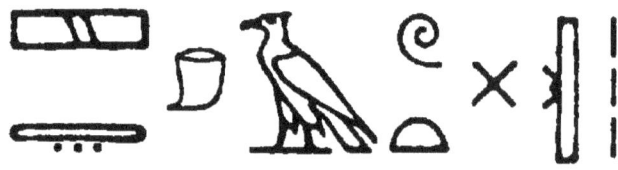

Shetaut means secret.

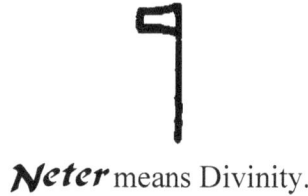

Neter means Divinity.

Question

The _____ is a symbol of Shetaut Neter, meaning the turning towards the light of truth, peace and transcendental harmony.

Who is Neter in Kamitan Religion?

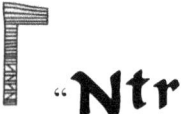

The symbol of Neter was described by an Ancient Kamitan priest as:
"That which is placed in the coffin"

The term Ntr, or Ntjr, comes from the Ancient Egyptian hieroglyphic language which did not record its vowels. However, the term survives in the Coptic language as *"Nutar."* The same Coptic meaning (divine force or sustaining power) applies in the present as it did in ancient times. It is a symbol composed of a wooden staff that was wrapped with strips of fabric, like a mummy. The strips alternate in color with yellow, green and blue. The mummy in Kamitan spirituality is understood to be the dead but resurrected Divinity. So the Nutar (Ntr) is actually every human being who does not really die, but goes to live on in a different form. Further, the resurrected spirit of every human being is that same Divinity. Phonetically, the term Nutar is related to other terms having the same meaning, such as the latin *"Natura,"* the Spanish Naturalesa, the English "Nature" and "Nutriment", etc. In a real sense, as we will see, Natur means power manifesting as Neteru and the Neteru are the objects of creation, i.e. "nature."

Sacred Scriptures of Shetaut Neter

The following scriptures represent the foundational scriptures of Kamitan culture. They may be divided into three categories: ***Mythic Scriptures***, ***Mystical Philosophy*** and ***Ritual Scriptures***, and ***Wisdom Scriptures*** (Didactic Literature).

MYTHIC SCRIPTURES Literature	Mystical (Ritual) Philosophy Literature	Wisdom Texts Literature
SHETAUT ASAR-ASET-HERU The Myth of Asar, Aset and Heru (Asarian Resurrection Theology) - Predynastic **SHETAUT ATUM-RA** Anunian Theology Predynastic Shetaut Net/Aset/Hetheru Saitian Theology – Goddess Spirituality Predynastic **SHETAUT PTAH** Memphite Theology Predynastic Shetaut Amun Theban Theology Predynastic	Coffin Texts (C. 2040 B.C.E.-1786 B.C.E.) Papyrus Texts (C. 1580 B.C.E.-Roman Period)[4] Books of Coming Forth By Day Example of famous papyri: Papyrus of Any Papyrus of Hunefer Papyrus of Kenna Greenfield Papyrus, Etc.	Wisdom Texts (C. 3,000 B.C.E. – PTOLEMAIC PERIOD) Precepts of Ptahotep Instructions of Any Instructions of Amenemope Etc. Maat Declarations Literature (All Periods)

---

[4] After 1570 B.C.E they would evolve into a more unified text, the Egyptian Book of the Dead.

NOTES:

What kind of text is Papyrus of Any?

The symbol of Neter is an Ankh? True/False

Neter and the Neteru

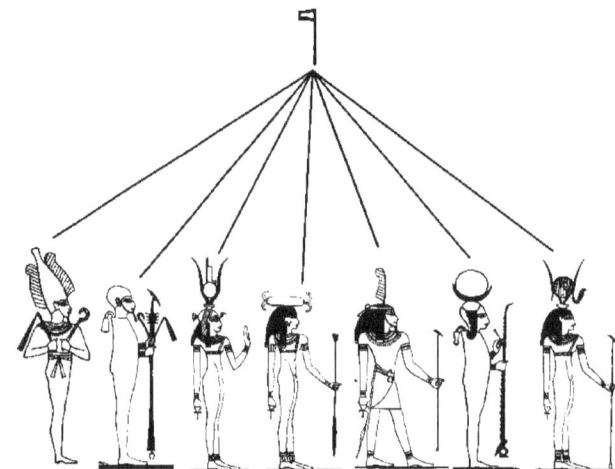

The Neteru (Gods and Goddesses) proceed from the Neter (Supreme Being)

As stated earlier, the concept of Neter and Neteru binds and ties all of the varied forms of Kamitan spirituality into one vision of the gods and goddesses all emerging from the same Supreme Being. Therefore, ultimately, Kamitan spirituality is not polytheistic, nor is it monotheistic, for it holds that the Supreme Being is more than a God or Goddess. The Supreme Being is an all-encompassing Absolute Divinity.

The Neteru

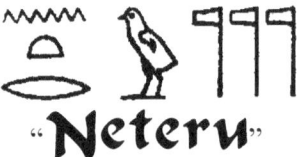

The term "Neteru" means "gods and goddesses." This means that from the ultimate and transcendental Supreme Being, "Neter," come the Neteru. There are countless Neteru. So from the one come the many. These Neteru are cosmic forces that pervade the universe. They are the means by which Neter sustains Creation and manifests through it. So Neterianism is a monotheistic polytheism. The one Supreme Being expresses as many gods and goddesses. At the end of time, after their work of sustaining Creation is finished, these gods and goddesses are again absorbed back into the Supreme Being.

All of the spiritual systems of Ancient Egypt (Kamit) have one essential aspect that is common to all; they all hold that there is a Supreme Being (Neter) who manifests in a multiplicity of ways through nature, the Neteru. Like sunrays, the Neteru emanate from the Divine; they are its manifestations. So by studying the Neteru we learn about and are led to discover their source, the Neter, and with this discovery we are enlightened. The Neteru may be depicted anthropomorphically or zoomorphically in accordance with the teaching about Neter that is being conveyed through them.

NOTES:

What is the meaning of the term "Neteru"?

The Neteru and Their Temples

Diagram 1: The Ancient Egyptian Temple Network

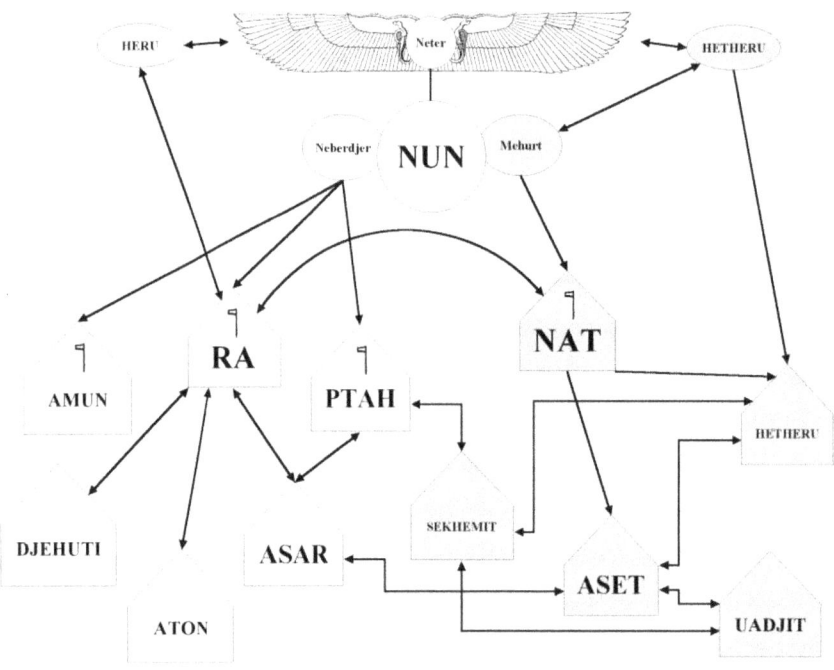

The sages of Kamit instituted a system by which the teachings of spirituality were espoused through a Temple organization. The major divinities were assigned to a particular city. That divinity or group of divinities became the "patron" divinity or divinities of that city. Also, the Priests and Priestesses of that Temple were in charge of seeing to the welfare of the people in that district as well as maintaining the traditions and disciplines of the traditions based on the particular divinity being worshipped. So the original concept of "Neter" became elaborated through the "theologies" of the various traditions. A dynamic expression of the teachings emerged, which though maintaining the integrity of the teachings, expressed nuances of variation in perspective on the teachings to suit the needs of varying kinds of personalities of the people of different locales.

In the diagram above, the primary or main divinities are denoted by the Neter symbol (⸠). The house structure represents the Temple for that particular divinity. The interconnections with the other Temples are based on original scriptural statements espoused by the Temples that linked the divinities of their Temple with the other divinities. So this means that the divinities should be viewed not as separate entities operating independently, but rather as family members who are in the same "business" together, i.e. the enlightenment of society, albeit through variations in form of worship, name, form (expression of the Divinity), etc. Ultimately, all the divinities are referred to as Neteru and they are all said to be emanations from the ultimate and Supreme Being. Thus, the teaching from any of the Temples leads to an understanding of the others, and these all lead back to the source, the highest Divinity. Thus, the teaching within any of the Temple systems would lead to the attainment of spiritual enlightenment, the Great Awakening.

NOTES:

teaching from any of the Temples leads to an understanding of the
_____

Listening to the Teachings

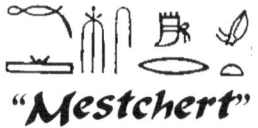

"Mestchert"

"Listening, to fill the ears, listen attentively-"

What should the ears be filled with?

The sages of Shetaut Neter enjoined that a Shemsu Neter (follower of Neter, an initiate or aspirant) should listen to the WISDOM of the Neterian Traditions. These are the myth related to the gods and goddesses containing the basic understanding of who they are, what they represent, how they relate human beings and to the Supreme Being. The myths allow us to be connected to the Divine.

An aspirant may choose any one of the 5 main Neterian Traditions.

- Shetaut Anu – Teachings of the Ra Tradition
- Shetaut Menefer – Teachings of the Ptah Tradition
- Shetaut Waset – Teachings of the Amun Tradition
- Shetaut Netrit – Teachings of the Goddess Tradition
- Shetaut Asar – Teachings of the Asarian Tradition
- Shetaut Aton – Teachings of the Aton Tradition

NOTES:

There are 3 main traditions in Shetaut Nete. True/False

The Anunian Tradition

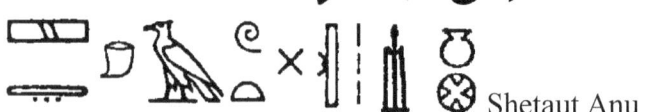 Shetaut Anu

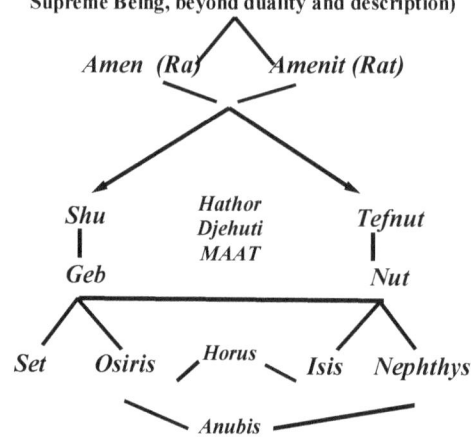

Below: The Heliopolitan Cosmogony. The city of Anu (Amun-Ra)

The Mystery Teachings of the Anunian Tradition are related to the Divinity Ra and his company of Gods and Goddesses.[5] This Temple and its related Temples espouse the teachings of Creation, human origins and the path to spiritual enlightenment by means of the Supreme Being in the form of the god Ra. It tells of how Ra emerged from a primeval ocean and how human beings were created from his tears. The gods and goddesses, who are his children, go to form the elements of nature and the cosmic forces that maintain nature.

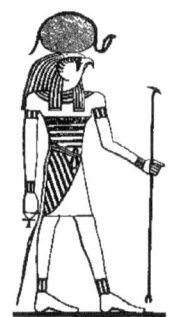

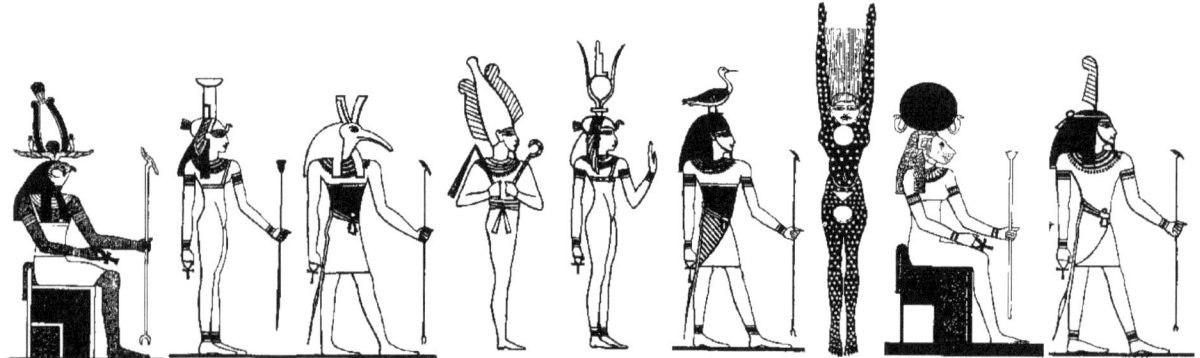

Top: Ra. From left to right, starting at the bottom level- The Gods and Goddesses of Anunian Theology:

Shu, Tefnut, Nut, Geb, Aset, Asar, Set, Nebthet and Heru-Ur

---

[5] See the Book Anunian Theology by Muata Ashby

Question

Ra emerged from a primeval _____ and how human beings were created from his tears.

The Memphite Tradition

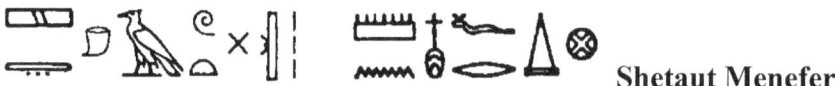 **Shetaut Menefer**

The Mystery Teachings of the Menefer (Memphite) Tradition are related to the Neterus known as Ptah, Sekhmit, Nefertem. The myths and philosophy of these divinities constitutes Memphite Theology.[6] This temple and its related temples espoused the teachings of Creation, human origins and the path to spiritual enlightenment by means of the Supreme Being in the form of the god Ptah and his family, who compose the Memphite Trinity. It tells of how Ptah emerged from a primeval ocean and how he created the universe by his will and the power of thought (mind). The gods and goddesses who are his thoughts, go to form the elements of nature and the cosmic forces that maintain nature. His spouse, Sekhmit has a powerful temple system of her own that is related to the Memphite teaching. The same is true for his son Nefertem.

Below: The Memphite Cosmogony.   The city of Hetkaptah (Ptah)

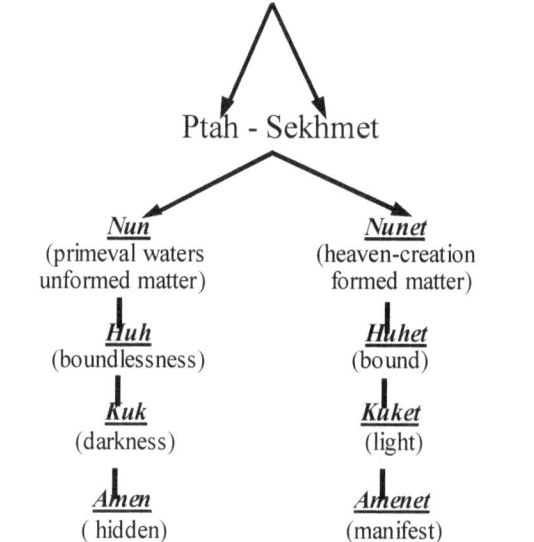

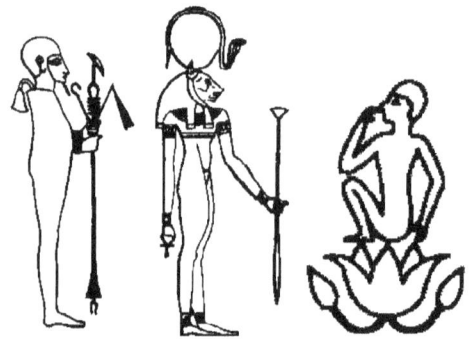

Ptah, Sekhmit and Nefertem

---
[6] See the Book Memphite Theology by Muata Ashby

Question

The gods and goddesses who are his thoughts, go to form the elements of _____

The Theban Tradition

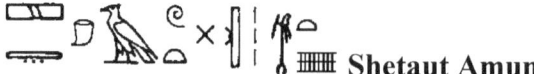 **Shetaut Amun**

The Mystery Teachings of the Wasetian Tradition are related to the Neterus known as Amun, Mut Khonsu. This temple and its related temples espoused the teachings of Creation, human origins and the path to spiritual enlightenment by means of the Supreme Being in the form of the god Amun or Amun-Ra. It tells of how Amun and his family, the Trinity of Amun, Mut and Khonsu, manage the Universe along with his Company of Gods and Goddesses. This Temple became very important in the early part of the New Kingdom Era.

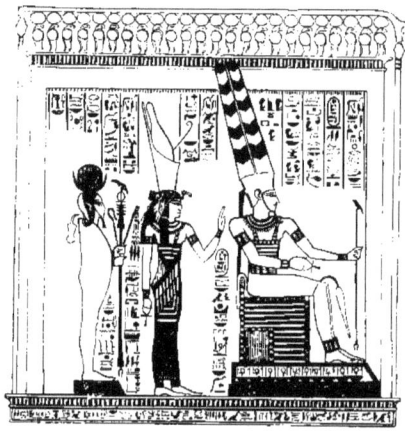

Below: The Trinity of Amun and the Company of Gods and Goddesses of Amun

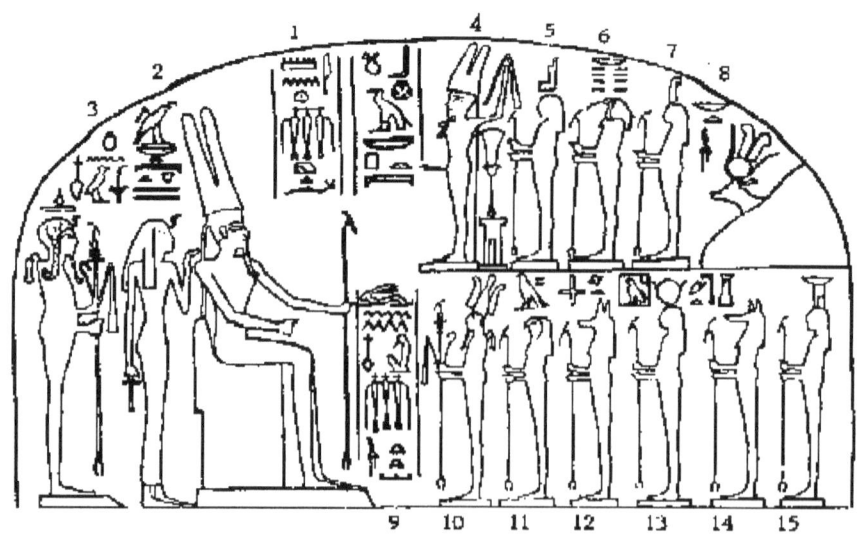

See the Book *Egyptian Yoga Vol. 2* for more on Amun, Mut and Khonsu by Muata Ashby

Question

In what period did the Temple of Amun become important?

The Goddess Tradition

Shetaut Netrit

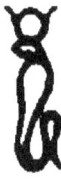

"Arat"

The hieroglyphic sign Arat means "Goddess." General, throughout ancient Kamit, the Mystery Teachings of the Goddess Tradition are related to the Divinity in the form of the Goddess. The Goddess was an integral part of all the Neterian traditions but special temples also developed around the worship of certain particular Goddesses who were also regarded as Supreme Beings in their own right. Thus as in other African religions, the goddess as well as the female gender were respected and elevated as the male divinities. The Goddess was also the author of Creation, giving birth to it as a great Cow. The following are the most important forms of the goddess.[7]

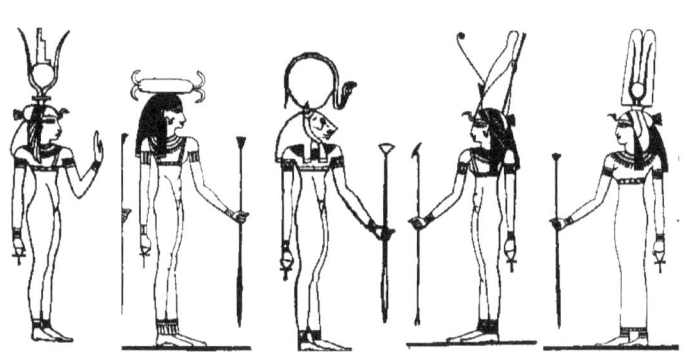

Aset, Net, Sekhmit, Mut, Hetheru

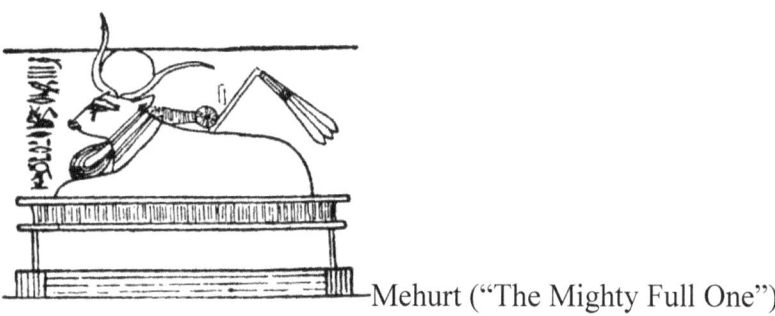

Mehurt ("The Mighty Full One")

---

[7] See the Books, *The Goddess Path, Mysteries of Isis, Glorious Light Meditation, Memphite Theology* and *Resurrecting Osiris* by Muata Ashby

Question

True or False

The goddess as well as the female gender were respected and elevated as the male divinities in Kemetic religion?

The Asarian Tradition

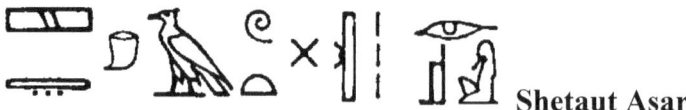 **Shetaut Asar**

This temple and its related temples espoused the teachings of Creation, human origins and the path to spiritual enlightenment by means of the Supreme Being in the form of the god Asar. It tells of how Asar and his family, the Trinity of Asar, Aset and Heru, manage the Universe and lead human beings to spiritual enlightenment and the resurrection of the soul. This Temple and its teaching were very important from the Pre-Dynastic era down to the Christian period. The Mystery Teachings of the Asarian Tradition are related to the Neterus known as: Asar, Aset, Heru (Osiris, Isis and Heru (Horus))

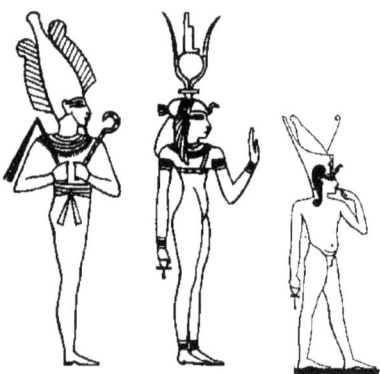

The tradition of Asar, Aset and Heru was practiced generally throughout the land of ancient Kamit. The centers of this tradition were the city of Abdu containing the Great Temple of Asar, the city of Pilak containing the Great Temple of Aset[8] and Edfu containing the Ggreat Temple of Heru.

---

[8] See the Book Resurrecting Osiris by Muata Ashby

Question

The tradition of Asar, Aset and Heru was practiced _____ throughout the land of ancient Kamit.

The Aton Tradition

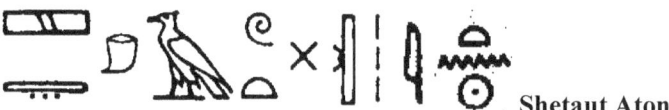 **Shetaut Aton**

This temple and its related temples espoused the teachings of Creation, human origins and the path to spiritual enlightenment by means of the Supreme Being in the form of the god Aton. It tells of how Aton with its dynamic life force created and sustains Creation. By recognizing Aton as the very substratum of all existence, human beings engage in devotional exercises and rituals and the study of the Hymns containing the wisdom teachings of Aton explaining that Aton manages the Universe and leads human beings to spiritual enlightenment and eternal life for the soul. This Temple and its teaching were very important in the middle New Kingdom Period. The Mystery Teachings of the Aton Tradition are related to the Neter Aton and its main exponent was the Sage King Akhnaton, who is depicted below with his family adoring the sundisk, symbol of the Aton.

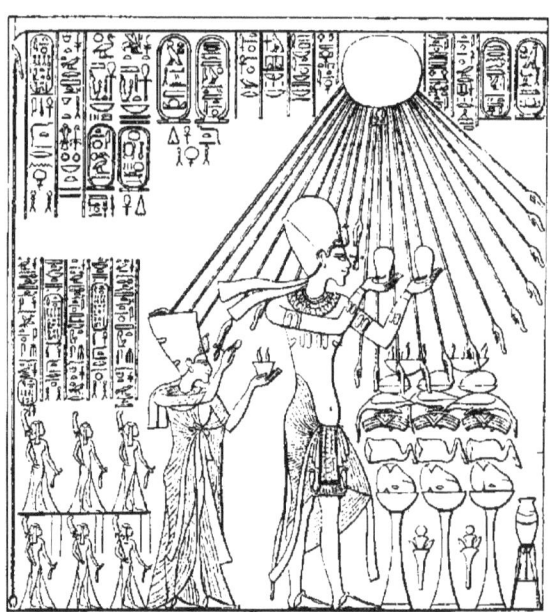

Akhnaton, Nefertiti and Daughters

Question

Teachings of the Aton Tradition are related to the Neter _____.

The Great Awakening of Neterian Religion

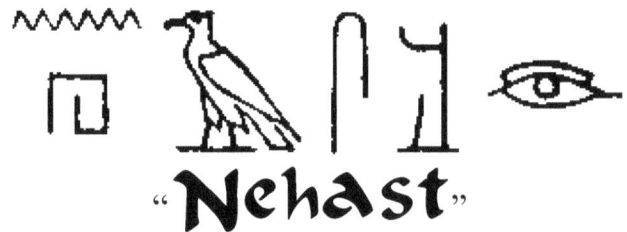

"Nehast"

Nehast means to "wake up," to Awaken to the higher existence. In the Prt m Hru Text it is said:

Nuk pa Neter aah Neter Uah asha ren
"I am that same God, the Supreme One, who has myriad of mysterious names."

The goal of all the Neterian disciplines is to discover the meaning of "Who am I?," to unravel the mysteries of life and to fathom the depths of eternity and infinity. This is the task of all human beings and it is to be accomplished in this very lifetime.

This can be done by learning the ways of the Neteru, emulating them and finally becoming like them, Akhus, (enlightened beings), walking the earth as giants and accomplishing great deeds such as the creation of the universe!

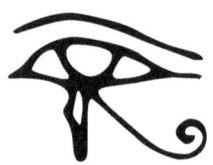

Udjat
The Eye of Heru is a quintessential symbol of awakening to Divine Consciousness, representing the concept of Nehast.

---

[9] (Prt M Hru 9:4)

NOTES:

Akhus, are _____ **beings.**

The goal of the Neterian disciplines is to discover the meaning of _____ _____ _____

The Teachings of the Temple of Isis and The Diet of the Initiates

While the general population was considered to be one of the most healthy groups of the ancient world, the spiritual initiates were required to keep even more strict dietary practices. The special diets of the ancient Egyptian initiates were a highly guarded secret as were the inner meanings of the myths which were acted out in the mystery rituals (**SHETAUT NETER**). For this reason, many of the special yogic practices which included a special diet and meditation were not committed to writing in an explicit fashion. Rather, they were committed to hieroglyphic form and carried on through the initiatic process. It was not until Greek historians and initiates into the Egyptian mystery schools began to write about their experiences that the more detailed aspects of the initiatic diets were available to a wider audience. The sect of Jews called the Essenes practiced an initiation period of two to three years and instituted purification diets and hygienic practices similar to those spoken about by Herodotus (484?-425 BCE) and Plutarch (46?-120 ACE). The Essenic health practices were presented in the Essene Gospel of Peace.

Plutarch, a student of the mysteries of Isis, reported that the initiates followed a strict diet made up of vegetables and fruits and *abstained from particular kinds of foods* (swine, sheep, fish, etc.) *as well as indulgence of the carnal appetite.* In the following excerpts Plutarch describes the purpose and procedure of the diet observed by the Initiates of Aset (Isis) and the goal to be attained through the rigorous spiritual program. This next excerpt should be studied carefully.

> *To desire, therefore, and covet after truth, those truths more especially which concern the divine nature, is to aspire to be partakers of that nature itself* (1), *and to profess that all our studies* (2) *and inquiries* (2) *are devoted to the acquisition of holiness. This occupation is surely more truly religious than any external* (3) *purifications or mere service of the temple can be.*(4) *But more especially must such a disposition of mind be highly acceptable to that goddess to whose service you are dedicated, for her special characteristics are wisdom and foresight, and her very name seems to express the peculiar relation which she bears to knowledge. For "Isis" is a Greek word, and means "knowledge or wisdom,"*(5) *and "Typhon," [Set] the name of her professed adversary, is also a Greek word, and means " pride and insolence."*(6) *This latter name is well adapted to one who, full of ignorance and error, tears in pieces* (7) *and conceals that holy doctrine (about Osiris) which the goddess collects, compiles, and delivers to those who aspire after the most perfect participation in the divine nature. This doctrine inculcates a steady perseverance in one uniform and temperate course of life* (8), *and an abstinence from particular kinds of foods* (9), *as well as from all indulgence of the carnal appetite* (10), *and it restrains the intemperate and voluptuous part within due bounds, and at the same time habituates her votaries to undergo those austere and rigid ceremonies which their religion obliges them to observe. The end and aim of all these toils and labors is the attainment of the knowledge of the First and Chief Being* (11), *who alone is the object of the understanding of the mind; and this knowledge the goddess invites us to seek after, as being near and dwelling continually* (12) *with her. And this also is what the very name of her temple promiseth to us, that is to say, the knowledge and understanding of the eternal and self-existent Being - now it is called "Iseion," which suggests that if we approach the temple of the goddess rightly, we shall obtain the knowledge of that eternal and self existent Being.*

Mystical Implications of the Discourse of Plutarch[10]:

1- It is to be understood that spiritual aspiration implies seeking the union with or becoming one with the thing being sought because this is the only way to truly "know" something. You can have opinions about what it is like to be a whale but you would never exactly know until you become one with it. God enfolding all that exists is the one being worthy of veneration and identification. This "knowing" of Neter (God) is the goal of all spiritual practices. This is the supreme goal which must be kept in mind by a spiritual aspirant.

2- In order to discover the hidden nature of God, emphasis is placed on study and inquiry into the nature of things. Who am I? What is the universe composed of? Who is God? How am I related to God? These are the

---

[10] Note: The numbers at the beginning of each paragraph below correspond to the reference numbers in the text above.

NOTES:

Fill in the blanks:

How should a spiritual aspirant think about the diet of the initiates as espoused by the temple of Aset and is it a realistic goal to be achieved?

You can have opinions about what it is like to be a _____ but you would never exactly know until you become one with it.

questions which when pursued, lead to the discovery of the Self (God). Those who do not engage in this form of inquiry will generate a reality for themselves according to their beliefs. Some people believe they have the answers, that the universe is atoms and electrons or energy. Others believe that the body is the soul and that there is nothing else. Still others believe that the mind is the Soul or that there is no soul and no God. The first qualification for serious aspiration is that you have a serious conviction that you are greater than just a finite individual mortal body, that you are an immortal being who is somehow mixed up with a temporal form (body). If this conviction is present, then you are stepping on the road to enlightenment. The teachings will be useful to you. Those who hold other beliefs are being led by ignorance and lack of spiritual sensitivity as a result of their beliefs. Thus, their beliefs will create a reality for them based on those beliefs. They will need to travel the road of nature which will guide them in time toward the path of spiritual aspiration.

3-4 The plan prescribed by the teachings of yoga is the only true means to effective spiritual development because it reveals the inner meanings of the teachings and it is experiential, i.e. it is based on your own personal experience and not conjecture. Otherwise, worship and religious practices remain at the level of ritualism only and do not lead to enlightenment.

5-7 The name "ISIS" represents "wisdom" itself which bestows the knowledge of the true Self of the initiate. In the Osirian Mysteries, when Set killed Osiris by tearing him into pieces, he was symbolically tearing up the soul. However, Isis restores the pieces of the soul (Osiris). Therefore, Pride and Insolence (Set-egoism) destroy the soul and Knowledge of the Self (Isis) restores it to its true nature. The Greek name for Aset (Isis) is supported by the ancient Egyptian scriptures. One of the names of Aset (Isis) is: *Rekhåt or Rekhit* meaning "knowledge personified" and "Isis-Sothis." *Rekh* is also a name of the God in the "duat" or Netherworld who possesses knowledge which can lead the soul to the abode of the Divine, thus avoiding the fiends and demoniac personalities of the duat which lead the soul to experience hellish conditions after death. The variation, *Rekh-t*, means Sage or learned person.

8- True spirituality cannot be pursued rashly or in a fanatical way by going to extremes. Yoga spirituality is a science of balance. It has been developed over a period of thousands of years with well established principles, which when followed, produce the desired effect of leading the initiate from darkness to light, ignorance to knowledge, an un-enlightened state to enlightenment.

9-10 The foods referred to are flesh foods (swine, sheep, fish, etc.), pulse, and salt. Indulgence in sexual activity has two relevant aspects. First, it intensifies the physical experience of embodiment and distracts the mind by creating impressions in the subconscious which will produce future cravings and desires. This state of mind renders the individual incapable of concentration on significant worldly or high spiritual achievements. Secondly, control of the sexual urge leads to control of the sexual Life Force energy, which can then be directed toward higher mental and spiritual achievement.

11- See #1.

12- There are two very important points in this line. Once again we are being reminded that good association or keeping the company of sages or other enlightened personalities is a powerful means to gain knowledge of the state of enlightenment. To this end, strive to keep good company in your family relations as well as non-family relations. Read uplifting books by the sages and the teachings of the masters. When you discover a more evolved personality, seek to maintain contact by reading their teachings and through correspondence. Do not debate with those who lack spiritual sensitivity. This form of interaction will weaken your mind. As Jesus said: *Cast not your pearls before swine, for they will trample them as they turn against you.* Trust in the Omniscient Divine Self, who knows past, present and future, who manifests as Nature to lead others on the path. Spread the teachings of yoga to those who are interested only or those whom you practice with. This kind of interaction will help you both to increase your understanding and generate a positive frame of mind.

Question

This state of mind renders the individual incapable of _____ on significant worldly or high spiritual achievements.

The second important point here refers to continuous reflection and meditation on the divine which is also expressed in the opening prayer in page one of this book: *"Give thyself to GOD, keep thou thyself daily for God; and let tomorrow be as today."* It implies that one's mind should be constantly remembering the divine and glorifying the divine in all things. It means not allowing the mind to develop attachments to the fleeting events of human life be they positive experiences or negative ones. It means not allowing the negative thoughts and feelings to lead you into a pursuit of illusory pleasures of the senses which will draw you away from divine awareness and realization. It means centering the mind on self-discovery and introspection at all times regardless of what your activities may be and those activities should be based solely on the principled of virtue, justice and order. This form of spiritual practice is known as "mindfulness" in Buddhism and Vedanta Philosophies.

Plutarch further reports that the Egyptian initiates:

> ...*strive to prevent fatness in Apis† as well as themselves*(1), *for they are anxious that their bodies should sit as light and easy about their souls as possible, and that their mortal part* (body) *should not oppress and weigh down their divine and immortal part...during their more solemn purifications they abstain from wine*(2) *wholly, and they give themselves up entirely to study*(4) *and meditation*(5) *and to the hearing* (3) *and teaching of these divine truths which treat of the divine nature.* † Bull which was kept as a symbol of Osiris and Ptah.

The following dietary guidelines for spiritual and physical health are derived from the above statement.

1- Preventing "fatness"- obesity. This issue is very important even for those without spiritual aspirations. Some people who are overweight claim that they are happy and content as they are. Some scientists claim to have discovered a gene in the human system which causes a propensity to become overweight. Once again, all of your body's characteristics are due to your past karmic history of experiences and desires, not only in this lifetime but in previous ones as well. Physical weight is like a physical object which is possessed. The more you have, the more you try to hold onto, and the more stress you have trying to enjoy and hold onto "things." Desires of the body such as eating have a grounding effect on the soul because they engender the desire to experience the physical pleasure of consuming food. Desires of the body as well as strong emotions such as hate, greed, etc., have the effect of rendering the mind insensitive to spirituality. Excess weight on the body causes innumerable health problems to arise.

You can change the future condition of your body by first mentally resolving to change it and then employing the self-effort in that direction while at the same time invoking the help of the Neters (cosmic forces - divine energies of God) to assist your quest for self-improvement. This will not be easy since the temptation of food is very great. It is related to the first energy center of the subtle spiritual body (Uraeus-Kundalini Serpent Power)[11] and it is a force which needs to be controlled in order to proceed on the spiritual path. As part of your spiritual program, begin controlling your intake of food gradually, on a daily basis. Even if you cut back a tablespoonful per day until you reach a level of intake which will support the normal weight for your body structure. Be especially watchful of yourself in respect to your habits. Do you eat out of habit, for pleasure or out of necessity? If it is out of habit or for pleasure, you must break the cycle by engaging in other activities when the desire arises. Do exercise, deep breathing, study, chant, call a fellow practitioner for support. The Serpent power will be discussed in detail in two future sections.

2- Natural wines and other naturally brewed drinks are acceptable in small quantities (for those still living worldly lives, but not recommended), however, you will notice that as you purify yourself, you will not be able to tolerate even a small amount of intoxicants. Distilled liquor is not a natural substance. It is processed into a potent form which is injurious to the body and is therefore, not suitable at all for use by those advancing on the spiritual path. The same applies to narcotics and all other "recreational" drugs. All of these distort the spiritual perception while damaging the physical body. No drug can

---

[11] see audio tape lecture Serpent PowerI - URAEUS YOGA: Workshop and Cleansing Meditation - I.

Question

Physical weight is like a _____ object which is possessed.

produce a high which can be compared to spiritual bliss. Therefore, resolve to leave all drugs behind and become intoxicated with spiritual feelings and aspiration.

3,4,5- Once again, the main format for spiritual education is:

 3- Listening to the teachings.‡
 4- Constant study and reflection on the teachings.‡
 5- Meditation on the meaning of the teachings.‡

‡Note: It is important to note here that the same teaching which was practiced in ancient Egypt of **Listening** to, **Reflecting** upon, and **Meditating** upon the teachings is the same process used in Vedanta-Jnana Yoga of today. See page 15.

Chapter 30B of the *Book of Coming Forth By Day* states:

This utterance (hekau) shall be recited by a person purified and washed; one who has not eaten animal flesh or fish.

Chapter 137A of the *Book of Coming Forth By Day* states:

And behold, these things shall be performed by one who is clean, and is ceremonially pure, a man who hath eaten neither meat nor fish, and who hath not had intercourse with women (applies to female initiates not having intercourse with men as well).

In the Mysteries of Osiris and Isis, Set represents the lower human nature and Heru (Horus) the Higher. Set kills Osiris and usurps the throne which rightfully should belong to Heru (Horus), Osiris' son. In various renderings of the characteristics of Set, it is stated that Set is promiscuous. Most interestingly, both Heru (Horus) and Set are vegetarians. Their favorite food is *lettuce*. Therefore, we are to understand that vegetarianism increases the potential for spiritual advancement and for the vital sexual force. With this understanding, it is clear that control of the sexual urge to conserve potential spiritual energy and purification of the diet are necessary practices on the spiritual path which enable the aspirant to achieve increased spiritual sensitivity. When practiced correctly, the conserved energy can be transformed into spiritual energy by directing it through the various energy centers in the body until it finally reaches the center of intuitional vision (Eye of Heru (Horus)-Udjat).

A most important point to remember when beginning practices for the purification of the body is that they should be implemented gradually, preferably under the supervision of an experienced person. If these changes result in an inability to perform your daily duties, then they are too extreme. The key to advancement in any area is steady, balanced practice. There must always be a balance between the practical life and the spiritual. In this way, spiritual advancement occurs in an integral fashion, intensifying every area of one's life rather than one a particular area exclusively. All areas must be mastered, secular as well as non-secular, in order to transcend the world process (illusion of time and space and the ego-self).

Since the physical body and all worldly attainments are changeable, fleeting and ultimately perishable, it would be wise to pursue a way of life which directs the mind toward understanding the Self and not to pursue health as an end in itself, but as a means to your own growth and spiritual evolution, which will continue even after the death of the your physical body if you have not attained enlightenment up to the time of physical death. The holistic development of an individual must be directed to achieving a state of consciousness which is not dependent on the physical body for peace and comfort. The body is an instrument which you have created through your thoughts to allow you to pursue the goal of enlightenment and thereby experience the fullness of life.

Question

The key to advancement in any area is steady, balanced _____.

The Recommended Daily Schedule for Yoga Practice

A practitioner of Yoga must be able to integrate the main practices of yoga into daily life. This means that you need to begin adding small amounts of time for Prayer, Repetition of the Divine Name (Hekau), Exercise (includes proper breathing exercise), Study of the Teachings, Silence, Selfless Service, Meditation, and Daily Reflection. This also means that you will gradually reduce the practices which go against yogic movement as you gain more time for Shedy.

Below you will find an outline of a schedule for the beginning practice of Yoga. The times given here are a suggested minimum time for beginners. You may spend more time according to your capacity and personal situation, however, try to be consistent in the amount of time and location you choose to practice your discipline as well as in the time of day you choose to perform each of the different practices. This will enable your body and mind to develop a rhythm which will develop into the driving force of your day. When this occurs you will develop stamina and fortitude when dealing with any situation of life. You will have a stable center which will anchor you to a higher purpose in life whether you are experiencing prosperous times or adverse times. In the advanced stages, spiritual practice will become continuous. Try to do the best you can according to your capacity, meaning your circumstances. If your family members are not interested or do not understand what you are trying to do simply maintain your practices privately and try to keep the interruptions to a minimum. As you develop, you may feel drawn toward some forms of practice over others. The important thing to remember is to practice them all in an integrated fashion. Do not neglect any of the practices even though you may spend additional time on some versus others.

Practicing spirituality only during times of adversity is the mistake of those who are spiritually immature. Any form of spiritual practice, ritualistic or otherwise is a positive development, however, you will not derive the optimal spiritual benefits by simply becoming religious when you are in trouble. The masses of people only pray when they are in trouble...then they ask for assistance to get out of trouble. What they do not realize is that if they were to turn their minds to God at all times, not just in times of misfortune, adversity would not befall them. As you progress through your studies you will learn that adversities in life are meant to turn you toward the Divine. In this sense they are messages from the Divine to awaken spiritual aspiration. However, if you do not listen to the message and hearken to the Divine intent behind it, you will be in a position to experience more miseries of life and miseries of a more intense nature.

Question

If your family members are not interested or do not understand what you are trying to do, what should you do?

Basic Schedule of Spiritual Practice

1a- Deep breathing, using the *proper breathing technique.*
1b- Alternate Breathing exercise (10 minutes in Am and in PM),
2- Prayer (10-30 minutes in Am* and in PM),

Opening Prayer:
O Åmen, O Åmen, who art in heaven, turn thy face upon the dead body of the child, and make your child sound and strong in the Underworld.
O Åmen, O Åmen, O God, O God, O Åmen, I adore thy name, grant thou to me that I may understand thee; Grant thou that I may have peace in the Duat, and that I may possess all my members therein...
Hail, Åmen, let me make supplication unto thee, for I know thy name, and thy transformations are in my mouth, and thy skin is before my eyes. Come, I pray thee, and place thou thine heir and thine image, myself, in the everlasting underworld... let my whole body become like that of a neter, let me escape from the evil chamber and let me not be imprisoned therein; for I worship thy name..

3-Exercise (10 minutes in am and before study time),
4-Repetition of the Divine Name in the form of your chosen hekau-mantra (10 minutes in am and in pm),
5-Meditation practice (10 minutes in Am, should be practiced after exercise, prayer and repetition of the Divine Name),

Closing Prayer after meditation or any spiritual practice:
I am pure. I am pure. I am Pure.
I have washed my front parts with the waters of libations, I have cleansed my hinder parts with drugs which make wholly clean, and my inward parts have been washed in the liquor of Maat.

6-Study of the teachings (reading 30 minutes per day),
7-Silence time (30 minutes per day),
8-Listening to the teachings: Choose an audio recording of a yogic spiritual preceptor and listen for a minimum of 30 minutes per day without any distractions if possible. If possible, go to a yogic spiritual center (Ashram, Wat, Temple) where teachings are presented by a qualified teacher of yoga wisdom. If this is not possible, form a study group wherein the teachings may be discussed and explored.
9-Selfless service (as required whenever the opportunity presents itself),
10-Daily reflection: Remembering the teachings during the ordinary course of the day and applying them in daily living situations- to be practiced as much as possible.
*(see Morning Worship and Meditation tape)

The suggested times given above are the minimum amount you should spend on daily spiritual practices each day. Whenever possible you should increase the times according to your capacity and ability. You should train your mind so that it rejoices in hearing about and practicing the teachings of yoga instead of the useless worldly activities. Follow this path gradually but steadily.

Once you have established a schedule of minimal time to devote to practices, even if you do 5-10 minutes of meditation time per day and nothing else, keep your schedule if at all possible. Many people feel that they do not have the time to incorporate even ordinary activities into their lives. They feel overwhelmed with life and feel they have no control. If there is no control it is because there is no discipline. If you make a schedule for all of your activities (spiritual and non-spiritual) and keep to it tenaciously, you will discover that you can control your time and your life. As you discover the glory of spiritual practice, you will find even more time to expand your spiritual program. Ultimately, you will create a lifestyle which is entirely spiritualized. This means that every act in your life will be based on the wisdom teachings (MAAT) and therefore you will not only spend a particular time of day devoted to spiritual practices, but every facet of your life will become a spontaneous worship of the divine.

NOTES:

Once you have established a schedule of minimal time to devote to practices, what should you do?

One should start your Spiritual Practice with a) exercise, b) prayer, c) breathing or d) meditation

What is the minimum time for meditation?

Introduction to The Kemetic Yoga of Wisdom

In the Temple of Aset (Isis) in Ancient Egypt the Discipline of the Yoga of Wisdom is imparted in three stages:

1-<u>Listening</u> to the wisdom teachings on the nature of reality (creation) and the nature of the Self.
2-<u>Reflecting</u> on those teachings and incorporating them into daily life.
3-<u>Meditating</u> on the meaning of the teachings.

Aset (Isis) was and is recognized as the goddess of wisdom and her temple strongly emphasized and espoused the philosophy of wisdom teaching in order to achieve higher spiritual consciousness. **The Yoga of Wisdom** is a form of Yoga based on insight into the nature of worldly existence and the transcendental Self, thereby transforming one's consciousness through development of the wisdom faculty. Thus, we have here a correlation between Ancient Egypt that matches exactly in most respects.

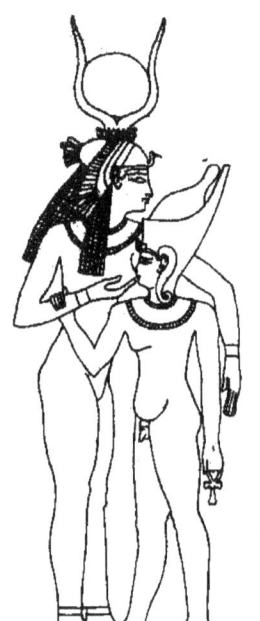

GENERAL DISCIPLINE OF THE TEMPLE OF ASET (PHILAE, EGYPT)

THE THREE-FOLD PROCESS OF WISDOM YOGA IN ANCIENT EGYPT

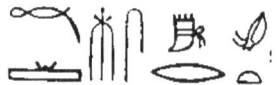

Fill the ears, listen attentively- Meh mestchert. -**Listening**

1 Listening to Wisdom teachings. Having achieved the qualifications of an aspirant, there is a desire to listen to the teachings from a Spiritual Preceptor. There is increasing intellectual understanding of the scriptures and the meaning of truth versus untruth, real versus unreal, temporal versus eternal.

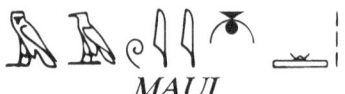

MAUI

"to think, to ponder, to fix attention, concentration" - **Reflection**

2- on those teachings and living according to the disciplines enjoined by the teachings until the wisdom is fully understood. Reflection implies discovering the oneness behind the multiplicity of the world by engaging in intense inquiry into the nature of one's true Self..

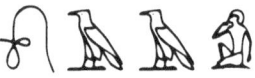

uaa

"Meditation"

3- The process of reflection leads to a state in which the mind is continuously introspective. It means expansion of consciousness culminating in revelation of and identification with the Absolute Self: Brahman.

NOTES:

Name the process in the practice in the Kemetic Yoga of Wisdom.

Introduction to The Kemetic Yoga of Righteous Action

GENERAL DISCIPLINE
In all Temples especially
The Temple of Heru and Edfu

Scripture: Prt M Hru and special scriptures including the Berlin Papyrus and other papyri.

STEPS IN THE PRACTICE OF RIGHT ACTION YOGA

1- Learn Ethics and Law of Cause and Effect-Practice right action
(42 Precepts of Maat)
to purify gross impurities of the personality
Control Body, Speech, Thoughts

2- Practice cultivation of the higher virtues
(selfless-service)
to purify mind and intellect from subtle impurities

3- Devotion to the Divine
See maatian actions as offerings to the Divine

4- Meditation
See oneself as one with Maat, i.e. United with the cosmic order which is the Transcendental Supreme Self.

Plate 1: The Offering of Maat-Symbolizing the Ultimate act of Righteousness (Temple of Seti I)

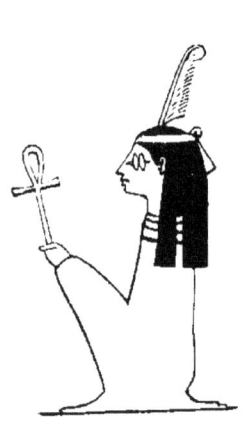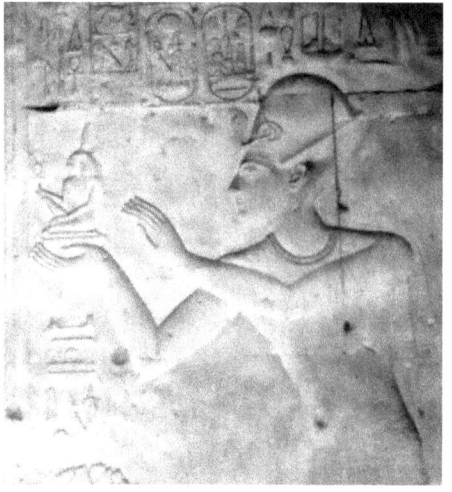

NOTES:

QUESTION:

What are the steps in practicing the Yoga of action?

How should a spiritual aspirant think about ego based feelings and how does the Action Path affect them as an aspirant transforms through time?

Ancient Egyptian Proverbs of The Action Path

"There are two roads traveled by humankind, those who seek to live MAAT and those who seek to satisfy their animal passions."

"They who revere *MAAT* are *long lived*; they who are covetous have no tomb."

"No one reaches the beneficent West (heaven) unless their heart is righteous by doing *MAAT*. There is no distinction made between the inferior and the superior person; it only matters that one is found faultless when the balances and the two weights stand before the Lord of Eternity. No one is free from the reckoning. Thoth, a baboon, holds the balances to count each one according to what they have done upon earth."

"MAAT is great and its effectiveness lasting; it has not been disturbed since the time of Osiris. There is punishment for those who pass over it's laws, but this is unfamiliar to the covetous one....When the end is nigh, *MAAT* lasts."

Kemetic Yoga of Action:

"No one reaches the Beneficent West* (Enlightenment) unless their heart is righteous by doing MAAT." *(the land of Osiris-heaven)

"Speak MAAT; do MAAT."

Yoga of Action implies acting according to the teachings of mystical wisdom (Maat) throughout your normal day to day activities. It keeps the mind occupied with thoughts which are uplifting to the mind. It is especially useful for calming the externalized-restless mind-set and redirecting thought patterns away from dwelling on mental complexes (worries) in order to allow the mind time to integrate its higher desire to overcome the difficulties through personality integration. Mental complexes will intensify rather than resolve if dwelled upon constantly. Many people have learned through experience that when there is a difficult problem which will still be there the following day, it is better to "sleep on it." When the clouds of egoism are no longer there, such as during deep sleep or in an advanced practitioner of yoga, the rays of the Self can shine through and illumine one's consciousness with *Hetep*. Again it must be emphasized that this experience of peace is not an all or nothing experience. It occurs in degrees. You may still find yourself feeling entrapped and agitated, but now, in addition to these ego based feelings, you have an increased sensitivity to the voice of wisdom within you. This is the voice which repeats a hekau, mantra or prayers and reflects on the nature of your true essence when the ego wants to tie the mind up with worries and imaginations. You may hear this voice repeating: *"I" am fearless. "I" have all the resources within me to withstand and rise above any situation. Even this seemingly impossible situation is in line with my attaining enlightenment, and it too, like the clouds in the sky blocking the rays of the sun, will pass away.*

In the beginning stages of practicing yoga when you are not very attuned to listening to your spiritual voice, you may not experience much peace. However, as you choose to listen to that voice more and more, and indulge in prayer, hekau and the other disciplines of yoga more than you indulge yourself in egoistic practices, you will notice within yourself a river of peace, faith, security and devotion which will eventually overflow and wash away all ego based emotions from your personality. This is the victory of Heru (Horus) over Set within your personality.

Question

Mental complexes will intensify rather than resolve if _____ upon constantly.

To the extent that you are able to control your temper, your inner war (between the Higher Self and the Lower) will not affect others around you, however, there may be an already established tendency to lash out at people around you. One should do one's best to sublimate this tendency and to remain focused on the negative and positive forces battling within oneself and work to establish Maat within one's self. This can be a difficult task when one is used to looking outside him/herself for answers and means to solve life's problems and blaming others (i.e. spouse, children, church, childhood, parents, country, political and religious leaders) for the occurrence of those problems. Situations can only affect you if it is in line with your karma for that to occur. Therefore, it is no accident or no one's fault or responsibility but your own regardless of what situation (good or bad) you may find yourself in. You may not be able to see how your actions of this life could have resulted in your current circumstance, but remember, these situations are occurring as a result of actions not only in this lifetime but previous ones. So your attitude towards dealing with all negative predicaments of life should be one of personal responsibility and forbearance. There is no need to feel bad or blame yourself or others. Blame and bad feelings are ego based viruses which infect the mind and further debilitate it. When you are typing and you make a mistake you don't spend a lot of time blaming yourself and having regrets about having made an error. You simply correct your error and carry on. The process with life should be similar. Pray for strength to endure and transcend the situation and put forth the effort to correct the error in your belief and thinking which predisposed you to have this situation manifest in your life. With patience and insight into the fact of your true underlying, boundless essence of your Higher Self, you can overcome all obstacles.

If you do not accept personal responsibility for your life, then you will never look to find that which may be in error in your thought processes and behavior which predisposed you to your experiences, and there will be no chance for you to improve your situation. If you do not learn the spiritual lesson that the situation is here to teach you, you are setting yourself up to have the experience repeat itself again. This is the nature of the karmic process upon which the world process is set up. These experiences are not meant to be painful or to make you bitter. Each of these experiences give you the opportunity to practice and secure spiritual qualities such as patience, equanimity, dispassion, detachment, universal love, freedom from resentment when persecuted or wronged and all the other precepts of Maat. In doing so, you learn to view every situation in your life as your path to enlightenment. In this way, performing your practical duties of life in a righteous manner becomes one and the same with your practice of spiritual discipline. Pain and suffering is a by-product of not living a life in harmony with Maat and with an awareness of your true essence.

The yoga of action also emphasizes the performance of selfless service, termed karma yoga. When one performs selfless service, the ego loses importance and therefore, its needs and cravings become powerless illusions which can no longer afflict the mind. The highest practice of karma yoga occurs in the state of enlightenment when there is no attachment to the fruits of actions. Work is performed in harmony with one's true nature without dependency on the results, be they good or bad from a practical standpoint. Right livelihood, the practice of making a living in such a way as to benefit oneself and all other beings is practicing Maat. Yoga of Action also implies a balanced movement and scheduling of time for spiritual discipline as well as other practical duties. Extremes are to be avoided because they also cause intensification of the mental complexes. The desired movement is relaxed and deliberate intensification of self-effort according to the capacity of the individual.

Question

If you do not learn the spiritual lesson that the situation is here to teach you, what happens?

Introduction to the Kemetic Yoga of Postures and Movements

Egyptian Yoga Exercise Thef Neteru:
The Movements of the Gods and Goddesses

The Yogic Postures in Ancient Egypt

Since their introduction to the West the exercise system of India known as "Hatha Yoga" has gained much popularity. The disciplines related to the yogic postures and movements were developed in India around the 10th century A.C.E. by a sage named Goraksha.[12] Up to this time, the main practice was simply to adopt the cross-legged meditation posture known as the lotus for the purpose of practicing meditation. The most popular manual on Hatha Yoga is the **Hatha-Yoga-Pradipika *("Light on the Forceful Yoga)*.** It was authored by Svatmarama Yogin in mid. 14th century C.E.[13]

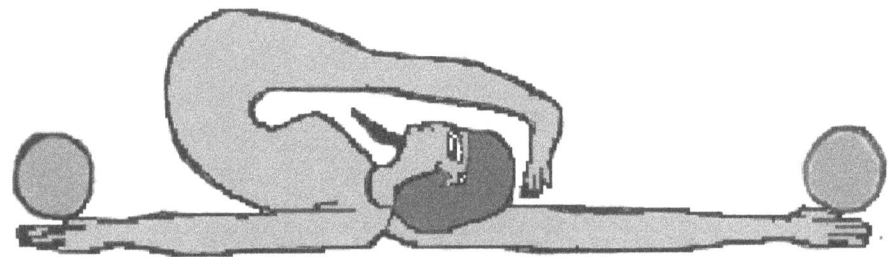

Plate 2: Above- The god Geb in the plough posture engraved on the ceiling of the antechamber to the Asarian Resurrection room of the Temple of Hetheru in Egypt. (photo taken by Ashby)

Prior to the emergence of the discipline the physical movements in India just before 1000 A.C.E.,[14] a series of virtually identical postures to those which were practiced in India can be found in various Ancient Egyptian papyruses and inscribed on the walls and ceilings of the temples. The Ancient Egyptian practice can be dated from 300 B.C.E 1,580 B.C.E and earlier. Exp. Temple of Hetheru (800-300 B.C.E.), Temple of Heru (800-300 B.C.E.), Tomb of Queen Nefertari (reigned 1,279-1,212 BC), and various other temples and papyruses from the New Kingdom Era 1,580 B.C.E). In Ancient Egypt the practice of the postures (called *Sema Paut* (Union with the gods and goddesses) or *Tjef Sema Paut Neteru* (movements to promote union with the gods and goddesses) were part of the ritual aspect of the spiritual myth which when practiced serve to harmonize the energies and promote the physical health of the body and direct the mind, in a meditative capacity, to discover and cultivate divine consciousness. These disciplines are part of a larger process called Sema or *Smai Tawi* (Egyptian Yoga). By acting and moving like the gods and goddesses one can essentially discover their character, energy and divine agency within one's consciousness and thereby also become one of their retinue, i.e. one with the Divine Self. In modern times, most practitioners of Hatha Yoga see it as a means to attain physical health only. However, even the practice in India had a mythic component which is today largely ignored by modern practitioners.

---

[12] Yoga Journal, {The New Yoga} January/February 2000
[13] **Hatha-Yoga-Pradipika,** *The Shambhala Encyclopedia of Yoga* by Georg Feuerstein, Ph. D.
[14] *The Shambhala Encyclopedia of Yoga* by Georg Feuerstein, Ph. D.

NOTES:

By acting and moving like the gods and goddesses one can do what?

Yoga postures began in India. True/False

The Yogic Postures Discipline

Most people believe that the practice of special movements or postures for the purpose of harmonizing the energies of the body, promoting health and a meditative mind began in India or China. Prior to the emergence of the discipline the physical movements in India just before 1000 A.C.E.,[48] a series of virtually identical postures to those which were practiced in India can be found in various Ancient Egyptian papyruses and inscribed on the walls and ceilings of the temples. The Ancient Egyptian practice can be dated from 300 B.C.E 1,580 B.C.E and earlier. Exp. Temple of Hetheru (800-300 B.C.E.), Temple of Heru (800-300 B.C.E.), Tomb of Queen Nefertari (reigned 1,279-1,212 BC), and various other temples and papyruses from the New Kingdom Era 1,580 B.C.E). In Ancient Egypt the practice of the postures (called *Sema Paut* (Union with the gods and goddesses) or *Tjef Sema Paut Neteru* (movements to promote union with the gods and goddesses) were part of the ritual aspect of the spiritual myth which when practiced serve to harmonize the energies and promote the physical health of the body and direct the mind, in a meditative capacity, to discover and cultivate divine consciousness. These disciplines are part of a larger process called Sema or *Smai Tawi* (Egyptian Yoga). By acting and moving like the gods and goddesses one can essentially discover their character, energy and divine agency within one's consciousness and thereby also become one of their retinue, i.e. one with the Divine Self. In modern times, most practitioners of Indian Hatha Yoga see it as a means to attain physical health only. However, even the practice in India had a mythic component which is today largely ignored by modern practitioners. The postures below are a few of those belonging to the Ancient Egyptian Mystery System. For more information on this discipline the book *Egyptian Yoga Exercise Workout Book* by Seba Muata Ashby

Some Postures from the Egyptian Yoga Movement System

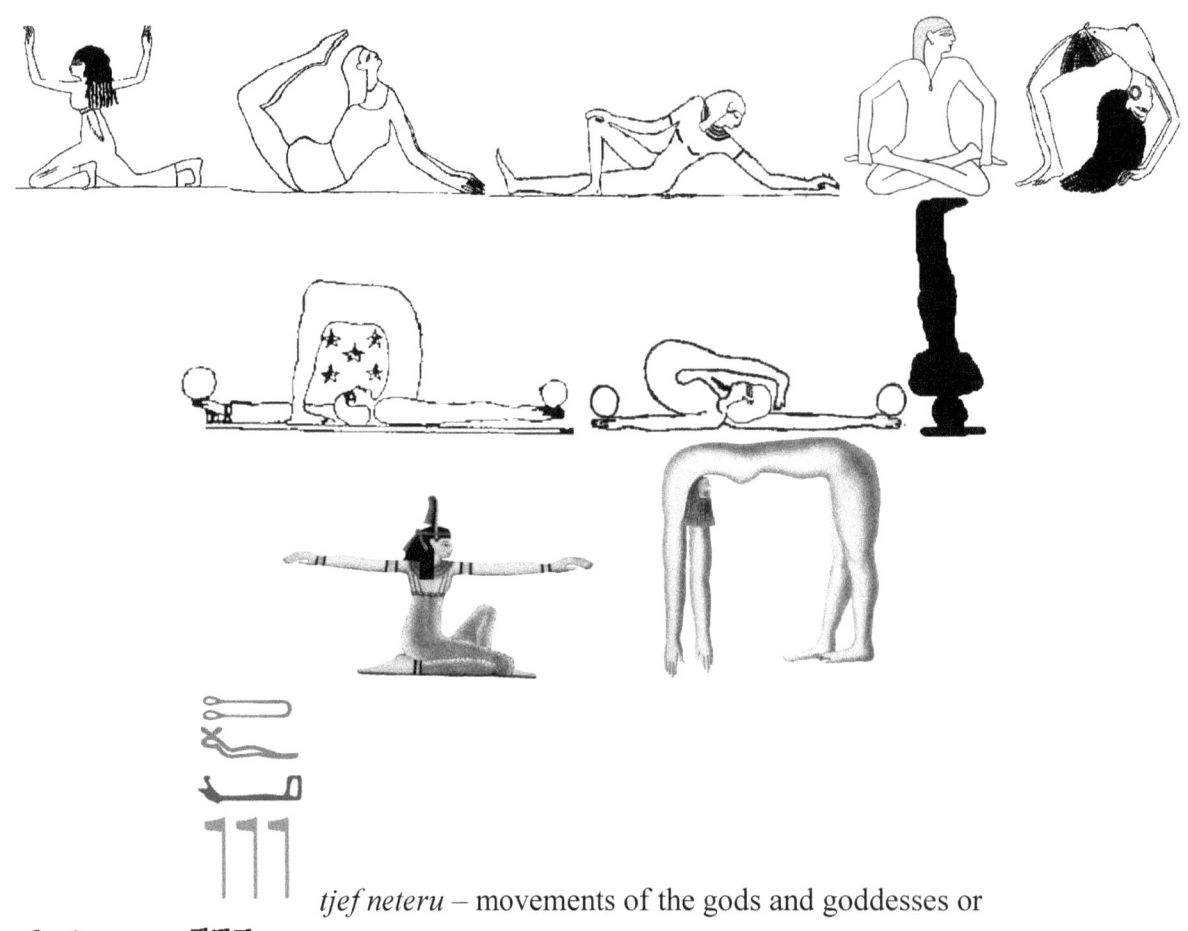

tjef neteru – movements of the gods and goddesses or

sma paut n neteru – Union with the gods and goddesses, the art of meditative movements in a ritual format to discover the power of the gods and goddesses within.

Question

In modern times, most practitioners of Indian Hatha Yoga see it as a means to attain _____ health only.

Physical Exercise:

"Her name is Health: she is the daughter of Exercise, who begot her on Temperance. The rose blusheth on her cheeks, the sweetness of the morning breatheth from her lips; joy, tempered with innocence and modesty, sparkleth in her eyes and from the cheerfulness of her heart she singeth as she walketh."

—Ancient Egyptian Proverb

Physical and mental health are the basis of spiritual health. Therefore, Yoga philosophy also includes the practice of special postures and exercises coupled with breathing techniques to promote the health of the mind and body. These exercises are psycho-physical in nature, affecting both the mind and body. These postures have an effect on one's mental attitude and physical health by stimulating, cleansing and balancing the various endocrine glands, organs and tissues of the body. Physical disturbance and preoccupation with physical illness may distract one's consciousness from higher, more sublime thoughts and aspirations. This branch of yoga is actually under the same discipline as meditation.

Recreation:

Recreation is a seldom discussed topic in philosophical treatises. It is usually seen as an "activity that is performed" in order to achieve some kind of regeneration of one's physical and psychological self. Also it is seen as a source of "fun" and excitement. The mind seeks to place itself in the most "pleasurable" environment or situations possible. From a deeper understanding of life and its purpose, the practice of many commonly accepted forms of recreation becomes inadequate because such activities have built into them, the elements of disappointment. Usually they are based on competition which pits individuals or teams against each other in a format that is designed to produce and promote conflict. Since the happiness to be derived is based upon "winning" a game, one is bound for disappointment since that cannot occur each time the activity is undertaken. If the times of disappointment are used for introspection, one will develop dispassion towards that which is illusory, painful and transient and seek to find that which is real, constant and truly pleasurable. A whole new world opens for exploration and true recreation in the spiritual realm.

True recreation is fully conscious, detached and peaceful. Only then is it possible to "feel" and appreciate the nature of one's being, of creation itself. The highest degree of recreation is therefore experienced at the point of enlightenment, when Heru (Horus)hood is realized. Here, every activity in life becomes "play." Life itself becomes a *"divine sport."* There develops a continuous blissful feeling which does not pass from moment to moment as with those who move from activity to activity searching for a thrill to make them "feel alive," but existence becomes eternity, right in the very present moment. As modern physics shows, time is only a mental concept people put on intervals of eternity. The only reason why we believe time actually passes is because our minds are always concerned with the past or future events and rarely with the present moment. Raising one's spiritual awareness means becoming alive in the present, the here and now. This has been elaborated in the section on Meditation.

Recreation becomes a means to re-create one's consciousness at every moment instead of a means to forget oneself and to pass the time. It allows you to be able to deal more effectively with life's problems rather than serving to distract you for a few minutes, hours or days. Many enlightened personalities from time to time indulge in recreational activities. The difference is that they do not identify himself with the pleasure or illusoriness of the event. As a therapeutic practice, he advocated recreation as a means to gradually adjust the mind and body to greater and greater levels of spiritual discipline. In short, a spiritual discipline does not consist in "giving up" recreation or pleasure; it consists in understanding that the pleasure comes from within, the Self, and not from the object or activity.

Question

Many enlightened personalities from time to time indulge in _____ activities.

Proper Breathing

Most people in the modern world do not know how to breathe properly. Most people (especially males) have learned to breathe by pushing out the chest in a "manly" or "macho" fashion. This mode of breathing is harmful for many reasons. The amount of air taken in is less and vital cosmic energy is reduced and becomes stagnant in the subtle vital energy channels, resulting in physical and mental diseases. The stagnation of the flow of energy through the body has the effect of grounding one's consciousness to the physical realities rather than allowing the mind and body to operate with lightness and subtlety.

"Belly breathing" or abdominal breathing massages the internal organs and develops Life Force energy (Ra, Chi or Kundalini). It will be noticed that it is our natural breathing pattern when we lie down on our back. Instruction is as follows: A- Breathe in and push the stomach out. B- Breathe out and pull the stomach in. This form of breathing is to be practiced at all times, not just during meditation. It allows the natural Life Force in the air to be rhythmically supplied to the body and nervous system. This process is indispensable in the achievement of physical health and mental-spiritual power to control the mind (meditation).

PROPER BREATHING: The way to promote health and control of the mind and emotions.

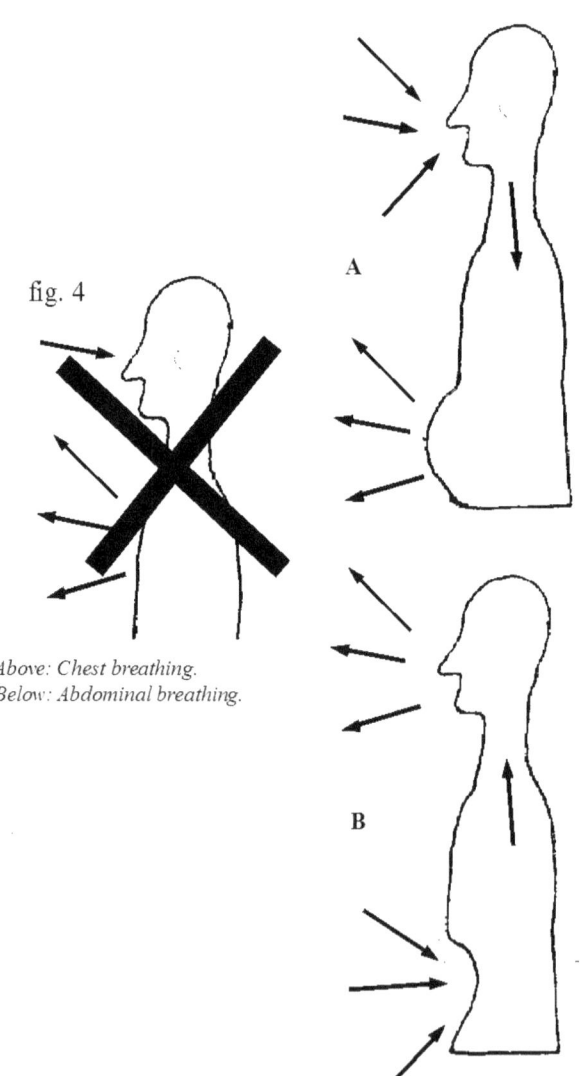

fig. 4

Above: Chest breathing.
Below: Abdominal breathing.

"GOD is life and through Him only Human kind lives. GOD gives life to men and women, breathing the breath of life into their nostrils."

"Be as the Sun and Stars, that emanate the life giving essence; give life without asking for anything in return; to be a sun, breath rhythmically and deeply; then as RA shall you be."

Ancient Egyptian Proverbs

NOTES:

The stagnation of the flow of energy through the body has what effect?

Introduction to The Kemetic Yoga of Meditation

KAMITAN HISTORY – 5 MAIN STYLES OF MEDITATION DISCIPLINES - Shedy

1. Arat Sekhem, The Path of the Serpent Power[15]
2. Ari Sma Maat, The Path of Meditation through Right Action[16]
3. Nuk Pu-Ushet, The Path of Meditation through "I Am" formula[17]
4. Nuk Ra Akhu, The Path of Meditation through Glorious Light system[18]
5. Rekh, The Path of Meditation through Wisdom[19]

3 stages in meditation

Concentration - Meditation – Superconsciousness
Mau — Uah — Syh

MAUI "to think, to ponder, to fix attention, concentration"	*uaa* "Meditation"	*Syh* - Ecstacy, religious	Swoon or subsiding during religious ecstacy - *Hed.*

---

[15] see book: The Serpent Power
[16] see book The Wisdom of Maati
[17] see book: based on the teachings of the Pert M Heru see book: Egyptian Book of the Dead
[18] see book: Glorious Light Meditation
[19] see book Mysteries of Isis

NOTES:

The Kemetic term 'uaa' means _____

How should a spiritual aspirant think about their capacity to control "Externalized consciousness" and their ability to rise above their conditioning of the past?

Introduction to Meditation and Hekau

"TO THINK, TO PONDER, TO FIX ATTENTION, MEDITATION"

INTRODUCTION TO MEDITATION

Up to now we have discussed continuous awareness of the Neter Neteru as a form of perpetual meditation practice throughout the day. Now we will explore the phase of meditation as a formal practice.

Meditation may be thought of or defined as the practice of mental exercises and disciplines to enable the aspirant to achieve control over the mind, specifically, to stop the vibrations of the mind due to unwanted thoughts, imaginations, etc. Just as the sun is revealed when the clouds disperse, so the light of the Self is revealed when the mind is free of thoughts, imaginations, ideas, delusions, gross emotions, sentimental attachments, etc. The Self, your true identity, is visible to the conscious mind.

The mind and nervous system are instruments of the Self, which it uses to have experiences in the realm of time and space, which it has created in much the same way as a person falls asleep and develops an entire dream world out of his/her own consciousness. It is at the unconscious and subconscious levels where the most intensive work of yoga takes place because it is here that the conscious identification of a person creates impressions in the mind and where desires based on those impressions develop. It is these desires that keep the aspirant involved in the realm of time and space or frees the aspirant from the world of time and space if they are sublimated into the spiritual desire for enlightenment. The desire to attain enlightenment is not viewed in the same manner as ego based desires; it is viewed as being aspiration which is a positive movement.

Externalized consciousness - distracted by egoism and worldly objects. ◄◄◄☉

The light of the Self (consciousness) shines through the mind and this is what sustains life. The flow of consciousness in most people is from within moving outward. This causes them to be externalized and distracted and lose energy. Where the mind goes, energy flows. Have you ever noticed that you can "feel" someone looking at you? This is because there is a subtle energy being transmitted through their vision (which is an extension of the mind). Those who live in this externalized state of mind are not aware of the source of consciousness. Meditation as well as the other disciplines of yoga serve to reverse the flow of consciousness on itself so that the mind acts as a mirror which reveals the true Self.

Internalized consciousness of a yoga practitioner. ►►►☉

Most people are unaware that there are deeper levels to their being just as they are unaware of the fact that physical reality is not "physical." Quantum physics experiments have proven that the physical world is not composed of matter but of energy. This supports the findings of the ancient sages who have taught for thousands of years that the reality which is experienced by the human senses is not an "Absolute" reality but a conditional one. Therefore, you must strive to rise beyond your conditioned mind and senses in order to perceive reality as it truly is.

"Learn to distinguish the real from the unreal."

Question

Those who live in this externalized state of mind are not aware of the source of _____.

Human beings are not just composed of a mind, senses and a physical body. Beyond the physical and mental there is a soul level. This is the realm of the Higher Self which all of the teachings of yoga and the various practices of meditation are directed toward discovering. This "hidden" aspect of ourselves which is beyond the thoughts is known as Amun, Osiris or Amenta in the ancient Egyptian system of spirituality.

Universal Soul
_____

↙ ↓ ↘

Mind and Senses
(Astral Body and Astral World - the Duat or Underworld)
_____

↙ ↓ ↘

Physical Body and Physical World

When you are active and not practicing or experiencing the wisdom of yoga, you are distracted from the real you. This distraction which comes from the desires, cravings and endless motion of thoughts in the mind is the *veil* which blocks your perception of your deeper essence, Neter NETER. These distractions keep you involved with the mind, senses, and body that you have come to believe is the real you. When your body is motionless and you are thinking and feeling, you are mostly associated with your mind. At times when you are not thinking, such as in the dreamless sleep state, then you are associated with your Higher Self. However, this connection in the dreamless sleep state is veiled by ignorance because you are asleep and not aware of the experience. In order to discover this realm you must consciously turn away from the phenomenal world which is distracting you from your inner reality. The practice of yoga accomplishes this task. Meditation, when backed up by the other disciplines of yoga, is the most powerful agent of self-discovery. The practice of meditation allows one to create a higher awareness which affects all aspects of one's life, but most importantly, it gives the aspirant experiential knowledge of his/her true Self.

Question

When your body is _____ and you are thinking and feeling, you are mostly associated with your mind.

What is Meditation?

Meditation may be thought of or defined as the practice of mental exercises and disciplines to enable the meditator to achieve control over the mind, specifically, to stop the vibrations of the mind due to unwanted thoughts, imaginations, etc.

Consciousness refers to the awareness of being alive and of having an identity. It is this characteristic which separates humans from the animal kingdom. Animals cannot become aware of their own existence and ponder the questions such as *Who am I?, Where am I going in life?, Where do I come from?,* etc. They cannot write books on history and create elaborate systems of social history based on ancestry, etc. Consciousness expresses itself in three modes. These are: Waking, Dream-Sleep and Dreamless-Deep-Sleep.

However, ordinary human life is only partially conscious. When you are driving or walking, you sometimes lose track of the present moment. All of a sudden you arrive at your destination without having conscious awareness of the road which you have just traveled. Your mind went into an "automatic" mode of consciousness. This automatic mode of consciousness represents a temporary withdrawal from the waking world. This state is similar to a day dream (a dreamlike musing or fantasy). This form of existence is what most people consider as "normal" everyday waking consciousness. It is what people consider to be the extent of the human capacity to experience or be conscious.

The "normal" state of human consciousness cannot be considered as "whole" or complete because if it was there would be no experience of lapses or gaps in consciousness. In other words, every instant of consciousness would be accounted for. There would be no trance-like states wherein one loses track of time or awareness of one's own activities, even as they are being performed. In the times of trance or lapse, full awareness or consciousness is not present, otherwise it would be impossible to not be aware of the passage of time while engaged in various activities. Trance here should be differentiated from the religious or mystical form of trance like state induced through meditation. As used above, it refers to the condition of being so lost in solitary thought as to be unaware of one's surroundings. It may further be characterized as a stunned or bewildered condition, a fog, stupor, befuddlement, daze, muddled state of mind. Most everyone has experienced this condition at some point or another. What most people consider to be the "awake" state of mind in which life is lived is in reality only a fraction of the total potential consciousness which a human being can experience.

The state of automatic consciousness is characterized by mental distraction, restlessness and extroversion. The automatic state of mind exists due to emotions such as desire, anger and hatred which engender desires in the mind, which in turn cause more movement, distractions, delusions and lapses or "gaps" in human consciousness. In this condition, it does not matter how many desires are fulfilled. The mind will always be distracted and agitated and will never discover peace and contentment. If the mind were under control, meaning, if you were to remain fully aware and conscious of every feeling, thought and emotion in your mind at any given time, it would be impossible for you to be swayed or deluded by your thoughts into a state of relative unconsciousness or un-awareness. Therefore, it is said that those who do not have their minds under control are not fully awake and conscious human beings.

Meditation and Yoga Philosophy are disciplines which are directed toward increasing awareness. Awareness or consciousness can only be increased when the mind is in a state of peace and harmony. Thus, the disciplines of Meditation (which are part of the Yoga) are the primary means of controlling the mind and allowing the individual to mature psychologically and spiritually.

Psychological growth is promoted because when the mind is brought under control, the intellect becomes clear and psychological complexes such as anxiety and other delusions which have an effect even in ordinary people can be cleared up. Control of the mind and the promotion of internal harmony allows the meditator to integrate their personality and to resolve the hidden issues of the present, of childhood and of past lives.

Question

The "normal" state of human consciousness cannot be considered as "_____" or complete.

When the mind has been brought under control, the expansion in consciousness leads to the discovery that one's own individual consciousness is not the total experience of consciousness. Through the correct practice of meditation, the individual's consciousness-awareness expands to the point wherein there is a discovery that one is more than just an individual. The state of "automatic consciousness" becomes reduced in favor of the experiences of increasing levels of continuous awareness. In other words, there is a decrease in daydreaming as well as the episodes of carrying out activities and forgetting oneself in them until they are finished (driving for example). Also, there is a reduced level of loss of awareness of self during the dreaming-sleep and dreamless-sleep states. Normally, most people at a lower level of consciousness-awareness become caught in a swoon or feinting effect which occurs at the time when one "falls" asleep or when there is no awareness of dreams while in the deep sleep state (dreamless-sleep). This swooning effect causes an ordinary person to lose consciousness of their own "waking state" identity and to assume the identity of their "dream subject" and thus, to feel that the dream subject as well as the dream world are realities in themselves.

This shift in identification from the waking personality to the dream personality to the absence of either personality in the dreamless-sleep state led ancient philosophers to discover that these states are not absolute realities. Philosophically, anything that is not continuous and abiding cannot be considered as real. Only what exists and does not change in all periods of time can be considered as "real." Nothing in the world of human experience qualifies as real according to this test. Nature, the human body, everything has a beginning and an end. Therefore, they are not absolutely real. They appear to be real because of the limited mind and senses along with the belief in the mind that they are real. In other words, people believe that matter and physical objects are real even though modern physics has proven that all matter is not "physical" or "stable." It changes constantly and its constituent parts are in reality composed of "empty spaces." Think about it. When you fall asleep, you "believe" that the dream world is "real" but upon waking up you believe it was not real. At the same time, when you fall asleep, you forget the waking world, your relatives and life history, and assume an entirely new history, relatives, situations and world systems. Therefore, philosophically, the ordinary states of consciousness which a human being experiences are limited and illusory. The waking, dream and dreamless-sleep states are only transient expressions of the deeper underlying consciousness. This underlying consciousness which witnesses the other three states is what Carl Jung referred to as the "Collective Unconscious." In Indian Philosophy this "fourth" state of consciousness-awareness is known as *Turia*. It is also referred to as "God Consciousness" or "Cosmic Consciousness."

The theory of meditation is that when the mind and senses are controlled and transcended, the awareness of the transcendental state of consciousness becomes evident. From here, consciousness-awareness expands, allowing the meditator to discover the latent abilities of the unconscious mind. When this occurs, an immense feeling of joy emerges from within, the desire for happiness and fulfillment through external objects and situations dwindles and a peaceful, transcendental state of mind develops. Also, the inner resources are discovered which will allow the practitioner to meet the challenges of life (disappointments, disease, death, etc.) while maintaining a poised state of mind.

When the heights of meditative experience are reached, there is a more continuous form of awareness which develops. It is not *lost* at the time of falling asleep. At this stage there is a discovery that just as the dream state is discovered to be "unreal" upon "waking up" in the morning, the waking state is also discovered to be a kind of dream which is transcended at the time of "falling asleep." There is a form of "continuous awareness" which develops in the mind which spans all three states of consciousness and becomes a "witness" to them instead of a subject bound by them.

Further, there is a discovery that there is a boundless source from which one has originated and to which one is inexorably linked. This discovery brings immense peace and joy wherein the worldly desires vanish in the mind and there is absolute contentment in the heart. This level of experience is what the Buddhists call *Mindfulness.* However, the history of mindfulness meditation goes back to the time of ancient India and Ancient Egypt. In India, the higher level of consciousness wherein automatic consciousness is eradicated and there is continuous awareness is called *Sakshin Buddhi.* From Vedanta and Yoga Philosophy, the teaching of the

Question

Philosophically, anything that is not continuous and abiding cannot be considered as real.

"witnessing consciousness" found even greater expression and practice in Buddhist philosophy and Buddhist meditation. Buddhi or higher intellect is the source of the word *Buddha*, meaning one who has attained wakefulness at the level of their higher intellect.

In ancient Egypt, this level of awareness was called *Amun*, "the witness" or "watcher." The practice of meditation has received much publicity due to the resurgence of the interest in Eastern religions. Perhaps the earliest recorded meditation practice and instruction comes from the teaching of the "Destruction of Mankind" which is inscribed in hieroglyphic text on the walls of a chamber in the tomb of king Seti I of ancient Egypt who lived between 2000 and 1250 BCE. It describes the words of power, visualization and posture elements of meditation and the procedure for practicing the meditation. This meditation text is presented in the book *"Egyptian Proverbs: Mystical Wisdom Teachings and Meditations"* by Dr. Muata Ashby

Tips for Formal Meditation Practice

Begin by meditating for 5 minutes each day, gradually building up the time. The key is consistency in time and place. Nature inspires us to establish a set routine to perform our activities; the sun rises in the east and sets in the west every day, the moon's cycle is every 28 days and the seasons change approximately at the same times of the year, every year. It is better to practice for 5 minutes each day than 20 minutes one day and 0 minutes the next. Do a formal sit down meditation whenever the feeling comes to you but try to do it at least once a day, preferably between 4-6 am or 6-8 pm. Do not eat for at least 2 hours before meditation. It is even more preferable to not eat 12 hours before. For example: eat nothing (except only water or tea) after 6 p.m. until after meditation at 6 a.m. the following morning. Do not meditate within 24 hours of having sexual intercourse. Meditate alone in a quiet area, in a dimly lit room (candle light is adequate). Do light exercise (example: Chi Kung or Hatha Yoga) before meditating, then say Hekau (affirmations, prayers, mantras, etc.) for a few minutes to set up positive vibrations in the mind. Burning your favorite incense is a good way to set the mood. Keep a ritualistic procedure about the meditation time. Do things in a slow, deliberate manner, concentrating on every motion and every thought you perform.

When ready, try to focus the mind on one object, symbol or idea such as the heart or Hetep (Supreme Peace). If the mind strays, bring it back gently. Patience, self-love and self-forgiveness are the keys here. Gradually, the mind will not drift toward thoughts or objects of the world. It will move toward subtler levels of consciousness until it reaches the source of the thoughts and there commune with that source, Neter Neteru. This is the desired positive movement of the practice of meditation because it is from Neter Neteru that all inspiration, creativity and altruistic feelings of love come. Neter Neteru is the source of peace and love and is who you really are.

Simple Meditation Technique

Modern scientific research has proven that one of the most effective things anyone can do to promote mental and physical health is to sit quietly for 20 minutes twice each day. This is more effective than a change in diet, vitamins, food supplements, medicines, etc. It is not necessary to possess any special skill or training. All that is required is that one achieves a relaxed state of mind, unburdened by the duties of the day. You may sit from a few minutes up to an hour in the morning and in the late afternoon.

This simple practice, if followed each day, will promote above average physical health and spiritual evolution. One's mental and emotional health will be maintained in a healthy state as well. The most important thing to remember during this meditation time is to just relax and not try to stop the mind from pursuing a particular idea but also not trying to actively make the mind pursue a particular thought or idea. If a Hekau or Mantra (Prayer) is recited, or if a special hieroglyph is meditated upon, the mind should not be forced to hold it. Rather, one should direct the mind and when one realizes that one has been carried away with a particular

Question

Do not eat for at least _____ hours before meditation.

thought, bring the mind gently back to the original object of meditation, in this way, it will eventually settle where it feels most comfortable and at peace.

Sometimes one will know that one has been carried away into thoughts about what one needs to do, or who needs to be called, or is something burning in the kitchen?, etc. These thoughts are worldly thoughts. Simply bring the mind back to the original object of meditation or the hekau. With more practice, the awareness of the hekau or object of meditation (candle, mandala, etc.) will dissipate as you go deeper. This is the positive, meditative movement that is desired. The goal is to relax to such a degree that the mind drifts to deeper and deeper levels of consciousness, finally reaching the source of consciousness, the source of all thought; then the mind transcends even this level of consciousness and there, communes with the Absolute Reality, Neter. This is the state of "Cosmic Consciousness", the state of enlightenment. After a while, the mental process will remain at the Soul level all the time. This is the Enlightened Sage Level.

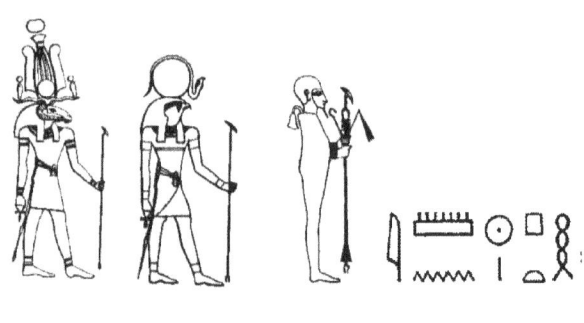

Amun-Ra-Ptah
The Holy Trinity

Simply choose a hekau which you feel comfortable with and sit quietly to recite it continuously for a set amount of time. Allow it to gradually become part of your free time when you are not concentrating on anything specific or when you are being distracted by worldly thoughts. This will serve to counteract the worldly or subconscious vibrations that may emerge from your own unconscious mind. When you feel anger or other negative qualities, recite the hekau and visualize its energy and the deity associated with it destroying the negativity within you.

For example, you may choose **Amun-Ra-Ptah.** When you repeat this hekau, you are automatically including the entire system of all gods and goddesses. Amun-Ra-Ptah is known as **Neberdjer,** the "All-encompassing Divinity." You may begin by uttering it aloud. When you become more advanced in controlling your mind, you may begin to use shorter words. For example simply utter: *Amun, Amun, Amun...* always striving to get to the source of the sound. Eventually you will utter these silently and this practice will carry your consciousness to the source of the sound itself where the very mental instruction to utter is given. Hekau-mantras are also related to the spiritual energy centers of the subtle spiritual body.

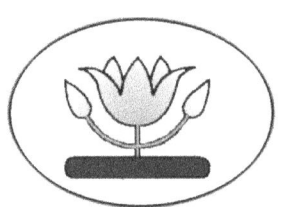

Question

When you feel anger or other negative qualities, what should you do?

Introduction to The Kemetic Yoga of Devotion

GENERAL DISCIPLINE-In all Temples
Scripture: Prt M Hru and Temple Inscriptions.

Steps in the practice of Devotion Yoga:

1- **MYTH:** Listening to the myths and divine glories of the various forms of the divinity (god or goddess) (in this case Asar)

2- **RITUAL:** Effacement of the ego through cultivation of love for the Divine (in this case Asar)
- Hekau (words of Power) Chanting
- Praises, Hymns, Songs to the Divine

3- **MYSTICISM:** Mystical union with the Divine – "I Am Asar"

God is termed *Merri*, "Beloved One"

Love and Be Loved
"That person is beloved by the Lord." PMH, Ch 4

Offering Oneself to God-Surrender to God- Become One with God:

Yoga of Devotion is the process of directing the mental energies (passion and love) to the Divine. It is a process whereby one uses one of the strongest emotions, love, to overpower mental afflictions and negative thoughts leading to union with the divine object of contemplation, one's Higher Self. In much the same manner that one rises above his/her problems and ailments when he/she falls "in love" with another person, so too when one directs feelings of love to the Higher Self, one is able to transcend problems and adversities in life. In addition, since human love is only a glimpse of cosmic love, imagine how much more powerful devotion to God can be in transcending the human condition. Devotion to God, also known as "Divine Love" is an effective way to produce mental health because it easily turns the mind towards the transcendental rather than towards the petty concerns of the ego. To practice Yoga of Devotion, throughout your day, feel that you are serving God when you are serving others, since all people are essentially the Self. In this way your mind does not become distracted by their personalities. When snowflakes fall, you do not become so distracted with their individual shapes that you fail to identify them as snow. Likewise, as intuitional vision of your all-encompassing nature dawns in your heart, you will be able to look beyond all the different sizes, shapes, sexes and colors of people and recognize your Higher Self as the basis for their existence.

43. Thou art Temu, who didst create beings endowed with reason; thou makest the color of the skin of one race to be different from that of another, but, however many may be the varieties of mankind, it is thou that makest them all to live.

Ancient Egyptian Hymn of Amun

"Souls, Heru (Horus), son, are of the self-same nature, since they came from the same place where the Creator modeled them; nor male nor female are they. Sex is a thing of bodies not of Souls."

—Ancient Egyptian Proverb from
The teachings of Isis to Heru (Horus)

NOTES:

_A_s intuitional vision of your all-encompassing nature dawns in your heart, you will be able to look beyond what?

What is the Kemetic term for Devotion?

When the mind is continuously directed toward the majesty and glory of God, the Neter (its Higher Self), the mind becomes imbued with that same glory and majesty. Thus devotion opens the way to the practice of the other disciplines of yoga (Yoga of Action, Yoga of Wisdom, Meditation) and these in turn lead to the experience of deeper devotion.

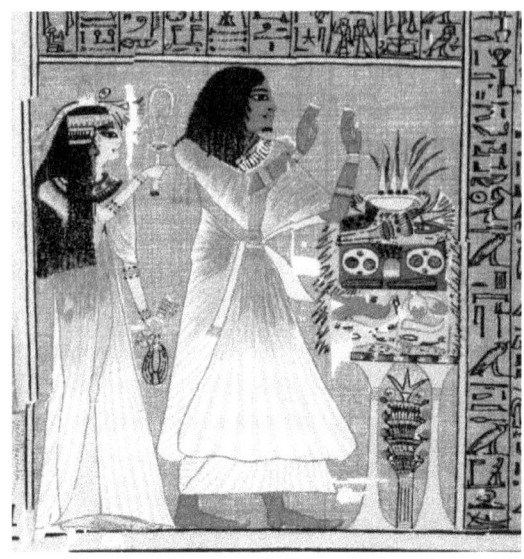

Ushet (devotion) Scene from the Papyrus of Ani- Ani in the Dua Pose- Upraised arms with palms facing out towards the Divine Image. His wife plays the sistrum to the Divinity (Asar).

Notes

THE RELATIONSHIP BETWEEN RELIGION AND YOGA

STEPS IN THE PRACTICE OF RELIGION

1 MYTHOLOGY	2 RITUAL	3 MYSTICISM
⬇	⬇	⬇
Learning the story of the god or goddess	*Ceremonies related to the myth*	*Meditation*
Devotion to the Deity: learning how to care for and love the Divine.	Right Living in accordance with the principles set forth by the deity in the myth.	Esoteric Wisdom about life and the spirit. Spiritual transcendence (Enlightenment)

TEXTS TO STUDY THE PATH OF RELIGION

A spiritual aspirant who feels a tendency towards approaching spiritual studies with a religious focus should concentrate on the following texts.

The Ausarian Religion and the Ausarian Trinity:
  BOOK: *Resurrecting Asar*
  BOOK: *Mysticism of Ushet Rekhat: Worship of the Divine Mother*

The Teachings of Anunian Theology and the Anunian Trinity:
  BOOK: *Anunian Theology*

The Teachings of Memphite Theology:
  BOOK: *Memphite Theology*

The Teachings of Theban Theology and the Universal Trinity
  BOOK: *EGYPTIAN YOGA VOL. 2: The Supreme Wisdom of Enlightenment-The Mystical Wisdom of Ancient Egyptian Theban Theology*

The books above are not exclusive of each other. They each relate to one another in order to show that while you may concentrate on a particular path, you may also integrate elements of others. Also, all of the Ancient Egyptian theological systems are related. They are a coherent expression of wisdom related to the Divine as it expresses in Creation. Thus, all the volumes introduce elements from the other paths and facilitate the practice of universal religion and yoga spirituality. It is important to understand that the religious path, when practiced in its three stages, leads to the same spiritual enlightenment which is possible through Yoga Mysticism. However, if religion and yoga are practiced at the lower levels only they will not yield spiritual enlightenment but dogmas and intellectualism.

Question

If religion and yoga are practiced at the lower levels only, what is the result?

How To Get Started On the Kemetic (Ancient Egyptian) Spiritual Path

WHAT IS THE NEXT STEP?

> "The lips of the wise are as the doors of a cabinet; no sooner are they opened, but treasures are poured out before you. Like unto trees of gold arranged in beds of silver, are wise sentences uttered in due season."
>
> -Ancient Egyptian Proverb

If after reading through the first portion of this volume you feel that the Kemetic Mystery Teaching is a path you want to explore then what is your next step? The next step if you choose to practice the mysteries is to learn more about the wisdom teachings and also the initiatic (yogic) disciplines to be practiced. You must become a pure vessel for the teaching so that you may be able to understand it. Otherwise the teaching will not have any effect. If you are in a dull condition even if Heru came to speak with you in a mystical vision it would do no good. You must first practice Maat. This is the first step on the road to purity of body, mind and soul. This is the path of virtue. Then you will be ready to fathom the glorious depths of the vast spiritual teaching and you will have the capacity to behold the magnanimity of the Divine which is all around as well as within you! As you purify and refine your spiritual search you will meet a preceptor who will show you the depths of the teaching and thereby also allow you do discover the depths of your own nature.

> "When the student is ready, the master will appear."
>
> -Ancient Egyptian Proverb

The Practice of Maat dictates that you should next practice the disciplines of Kemetic Yoga. So what is Kemetic Yoga? The following section provides you a basic introduction.

The Paths of Yoga

The Egyptian Yoga Book Series is written in such a way as to provide for the needs of various personality types. As stated earlier there are four major personality types among human beings. When those aspects are harmonized and when the person grows by developing each of those aspects it is said that they are practicing Integral Yoga. Therefore, the Egyptian Yoga Book Series has been put together in such a fashion as to offer every individual a specific discipline as well as an integrated method to practice all forms of yoga while at the same time advancing through the three stages of religion. The Asarian Resurrection, the Teachings of Memphite Theology and the Teachings of Theban Theology are the heart of Ancient Egyptian Religion and Yoga. It is from these teachings that the various path to spiritual realization emerge.

The Paths of Yoga may be seen as the four sides of a pyramid. They all lead to the same point at the apex. The eye symbolizes the attainment of Self-knowledge, Spiritual Enlightenment. So if you are interested in a religious yogic experience, understanding the mystical symbolism of the characters in Ancient Egyptian mythology and the Devotional path of Yoga the books *Resurrecting Osiris, Egyptian Yoga Vol. 2 The Supreme Wisdom of Enlightenment-Path of Amun, Mysticism of Ushet Rekhat: Worship of the Divine Mother* and *The Path of Divine Love* will be your emphasis in the study and practice of the teachings. If you are interested in an intellectual experience of enlightening the mind by eradicating ignorance through reason and reflection, and to leading yourself to greater and greater subtlety and spiritual enlightenment and the Wisdom path of Yoga, the books *Egyptian Yoga Vol. 1 The Philosophy of Enlightenment, The Philosophy of Enlightenment, The Hidden Properties of Matter, Mysteries of Isis,* will be your emphasis in the study and practice of the teachings.

NOTES:

The Egyptian Yoga Book Series has been put together in such a fashion as to offer what?

How should an aspirant think about their prospects to follow an integral path of *Sema Tawi* -Kemetic Yoga?

The 4 aspects of the personality are _____, _____, _____, _____ ?

If you are interested in the path of righteous action and the selfless-service path of Yoga, the books *Introduction to Maat Philosophy, Egyptian Yoga Vol 2. The Supreme Wisdom of Enlightenment* and *Egyptian Proverbs* will be your emphasis in the study and practice of the teachings. Also the book *Healing the Criminal Heart: Introduction to Maat Philosophy, Yoga and Spiritual Redemption Through the Path of Virtue* is good for anyone who would like to gain insight into the nature of sin (egoism) and how the practice of Maat Philosophy can lead anyone to a complete transformation, forgiveness and spiritual realization, regardless of their past.

If you are interested in the path of meditation and the Yoga of Meditation, the books *Meditation: The Ancient Egyptian Path to Enlightenment, Initiation Into Egyptian Yoga: The Secrets of Shedy, The Egyptian Yoga Exercise Workout Book* and *The Blooming Lotus of Divine Love* will be your emphasis in the study and practice of the teachings.

If you are interested in the path of Tantrism which involves discovering and developing the inner Life Force energies in order to direct them towards psychic powers and expansion in consciousness leading to union with the Divine and the Yoga of The Serpent Power and the Yoga of Tantra, the books *The Serpent Power: The Ancient Egyptian Wisdom of the Inner Life Force, Sacred Sexuality Egyptian Tantra Yoga: The Art of Sex Sublimation and Universal Consciousness* and *The Egyptian Yoga Postures of te Gods and Goddesses Book* will be your emphasis in the study and practice of the teachings.

For more on the path of Mystical Religion see the books *African Religion Vol 4 Asarian Theology* and *Egyptian Yoga Volume 2,* and *African Religion Vol 3 Memphite Theology.*

Integral Path: blending the disciplines to meet the needs of your personality

The personality of every human being is somewhat different from every other. However the Sages have identified four basic factors which are common to all human personalities. These factors are: Emotion, Reason, Action and Will. This means that in order for a human being to evolve, all aspects of the personality must progress in an integral fashion. Therefore, four major forms of Yoga disciplines have evolved and each is specifically designed to promote a positive movement in one of the areas of personality. The Yoga of Devotional Love enhances and harnesses the emotional aspect in a human personality and directs it towards the Higher Self. The Yoga of Wisdom enhances and harnesses the reasoning aspect in a human personality and directs it towards the Higher Self. The Yoga of Action enhances and harnesses the movement and behavior aspect in a human personality and directs it towards the Higher Self. The Yoga of Meditation enhances and harnesses the willing aspect in a human personality and directs it towards the Higher Self.

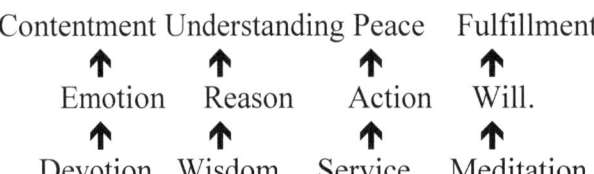

Contentment Understanding Peace Fulfillment
↑ ↑ ↑ ↑
Emotion Reason Action Will.
↑ ↑ ↑ ↑
Devotion Wisdom Service Meditation

Thus, Yoga is a discipline of spiritual living which transforms every aspect of personality in an integral fashion, leaving no aspect of a human being behind. This is important because an unbalanced movement will lead to frustration, more ignorance, more distraction and more illusions leading away from the Higher Self. For example, if a person develops the reasoning aspect of personality he or she may come to believe that they have discovered the Higher Self, however when it comes to dealing with some problem of life, such as the death of a loved one, they cannot control their emotions, or if they are tempted to do something unrighteous, such as smoking, they cannot control their actions and have no will power to resist. The vision of Integral Yoga is a lofty goal which every human being can achieve with the proper guidance, self-effort and repeated practice. There is a very simple philosophy behind Integral Yoga. During the course of the day you may find yourself doing various activities. Sometimes you will be quiet, at other times you will be busy at work, at other times you might be interacting with people, etc. Integral Yoga gives you the opportunity to practice yoga at all times. When you have quiet time you can practice meditation, when at work you can practice righteous action and selfless service, when you have leisure time you can study and reflect on the teachings and when you feel the

NOTES:

The Yoga of Devotional Love enhances and harnesses the _____ aspect of the personality.

Describe the 4 main paths of yoga practice.

sentiment of love for a person or object you like you can practice remembering the Divine Self who made it possible for you to experience the company of those personalities or the opportunity to acquire those objects. From a higher perspective you can practice reflecting on how the people and objects in creation are expressions of the Divine and this movement will lead you to a spontaneous and perpetual state of ecstasy, peace and bliss which are the hallmarks of spiritual enlightenment. The purpose of Integral Yoga is therefore to promote integration of the whole personality of a human being which will lead to complete spiritual enlightenment. Thus Integral Yoga should be understood as the most effective method to practice mystical spirituality.

    The important point to remember is that all aspects of yoga can and should be used in an integral fashion to generate an efficient and harmonized spiritual movement in the practitioner. Therefore, while there may be an area of special emphasis, other elements are bound to become part of the yoga program as needed. For example, while a yogin may place emphasis on the Yoga of Wisdom, they may also practice Devotional Yoga and Meditation Yoga along with the wisdom studies. Further, it must be understood that as you practice one path of yoga, others will also develop automatically. For example, as you practice the Yoga of Wisdom your faith will increase or as you practice the Yoga of Devotion your wisdom will increase. If this movement does not occur your wisdom alone will by dry intellectualism or your faith alone will be blind faith. So when we speak of wisdom here we are referring to wisdom gained through experience or intuitional wisdom and not intellectual wisdom which is speculative. If you do not practice the teachings through the Yoga of Action, your wisdom and faith will be shallow because you have not experienced the truth of the teachings and allowed yourself the opportunity to test your knowledge and faith. If you do not have introspection and faith, your wisdom and actions you will externalized, agitated and distracted. Your spiritual realization will be insubstantial, weak and lacking stability. You will not be able to meet the challenges of life nor will you be able to discover true spiritual realization in this lifetime or even after death. Therefore, the integral path of yoga, with proper guidance, is the most secure method to achieve genuine spiritual enlightenment. See chart of spiritual paths (below).

Question

Integral Yoga gives you the opportunity to practice Yoga at all times. True/False.

Integral (Wholistic) Yoga

The Process of Personality Integration

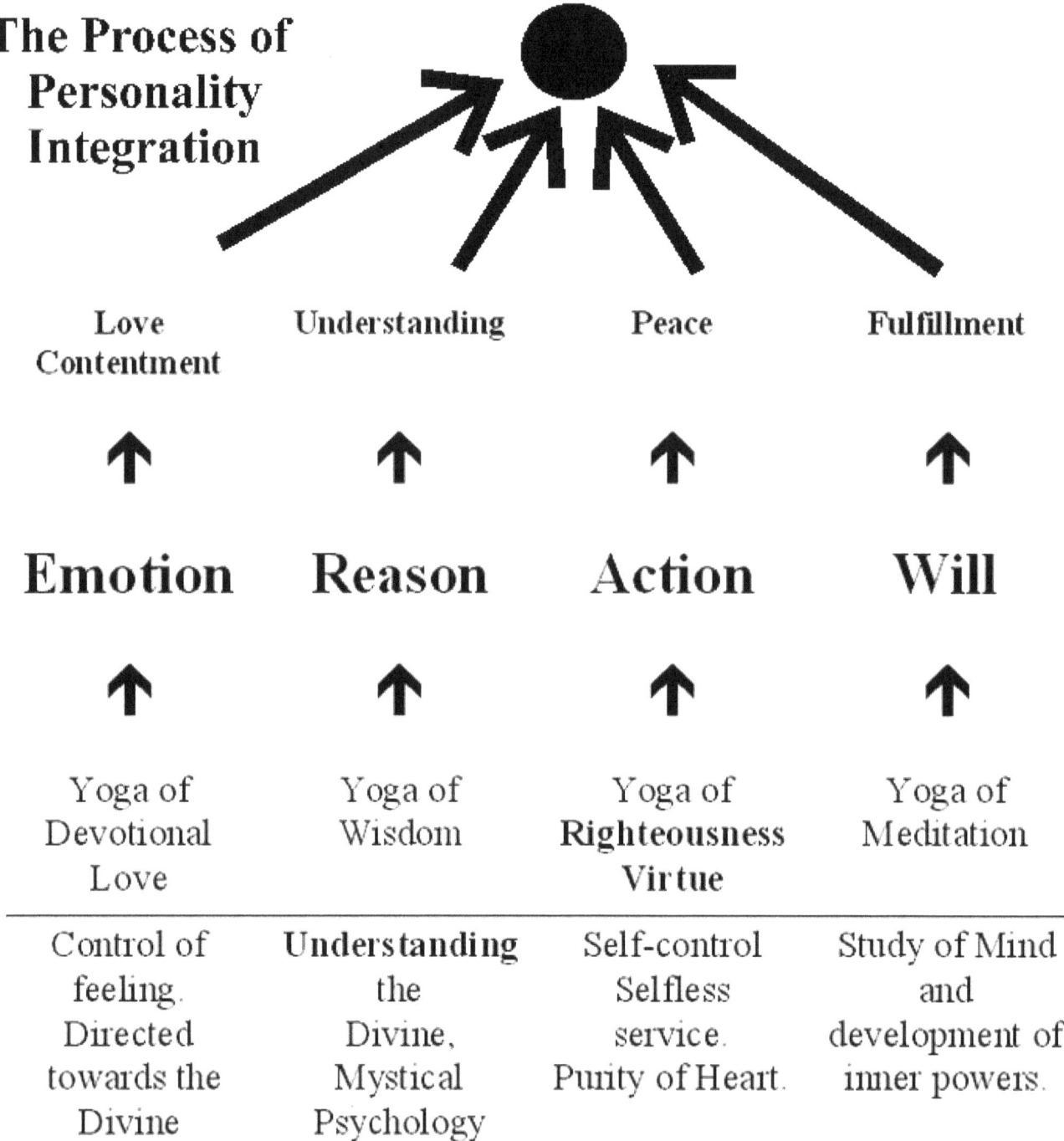

Love Contentment	Understanding	Peace	Fulfillment
↑	↑	↑	↑
Emotion	**Reason**	**Action**	**Will**
↑	↑	↑	↑
Yoga of Devotional Love	Yoga of Wisdom	Yoga of **Righteousness Virtue**	Yoga of Meditation
Control of feeling. Directed towards the Divine	Understanding the Divine, Mystical Psychology	Self-control Selfless service. Purity of Heart.	Study of Mind and development of inner powers.

The Paths of Yoga

NOTES:

Topic The Process of Yoga? a) Integral

The Yoga of Meditation controls the feeling directed towards the Divine. True/False.

PURPOSE OF THE INTEGRAL YOGIC DISCIPLINES

To Enlighten the Intellect	To Enlighten the Emotions	To Enlighten the Body	To Enlighten the Unconscious Mind
⬇	⬇	⬇	⬇
Yoga of Wisdom	Yoga of Devotional Love	Yoga of Right Action	Yoga of Formal Meditation

Study and Reflection

Listening should be followed by reflection upon the teachings. However, sometimes questions arise. At this time the aspirant should articulate the question and ask. Asking questions is the duty of an aspirant because it opens the door to understanding. However, once a question has been answered the answer should be reflected upon and assimilated. Sometimes an agitated mind is already thinking of the next question or a follow-up without taking care to understand the answer to the first question. This will lead to confusion. Reflection is an art and it is best carried out in silence, not only of the mouth but of the mind as well. So an aspirant should learn to ask questions and then to reflect upon them and living in accordance with the new understanding. In this manner the mind will be transformed.

"Seek to perform your duties to your highest ability, this way your actions will be blameless."
Ancient Egyptian Proverbs

There is one critical factor that every aspirant needs to understand. That is, how to balance the day to day reality with the teaching that is being learned. In the teaching you will learn how to transcend the world but this does not mean that the world is to be left behind. If you have responsibilities to maintain yourself or your family, like a job or like taking care of your children, spouse, etc. you must fulfill those responsibilities. You have gotten yourself into them by your past ignorance and you must get out of them by fulfilling your responsibility (Wisdom and righteous action). This means that if before you began studying the teaching and learning how to simplify your life and that you don't need a spouse to make yourself happy this does not mean that you go out and get a divorce. You need to fulfill your part of the relationship and understand the deeper meaning of relationships (See *Egyptian Tantra Yoga*). If you discover that you don't need a new expensive car you cannot just stop the payments. These actions would be against Maat. You must see the relationship to its conclusion even as you grow in enlightenment. You must make the car payments until you sell it and get out of dept properly. Leave nothing undone every day so that your mind may have peace everyday to study and practice the teachings and so that at the time of your death you will not be held back (reincarnation) due to unfinished business. The day to day activities have been created for your benefit. The people that you meet and the responsibilities you need to fulfill daily are the means by which the Divine Self is allowing you to work out the mystery of life by putting the teaching into action. Therefore, do not reject this gift of time, life, and activity. There should not be a contradiction between your inner life and your outer life. This contradiction is eradicated by the study of the teachings with the proper guidance. Therefore, attend as many classes as possible and listen to the tapes as often as possible. Use it wisely and you will see how your inner life and your activities in the world will work hand and hand to lead you to enlightenment. (See *The Wisdom of Maati*)

"The nature of the body is to take delight and pleasure in complexity;
the way of truth is that of simplicity."
Ancient Egyptian Proverbs

NOTES:

What is the one critical factor every aspirant should understand?

The key to success in allowing the inner gifts of the soul and the knowledge that leads to self-discovery to unfold is simplicity. Simplicity relates not only to the teachings but to one's practical life. How many possessions do you have and how many do you really need? How many car payments, stereos, or jewelry do you have? How much concern do you have about the body? What pleasures are you running after? What are you trying to accomplish in life and why? Are you trying to get rich, famous, to be voted the sexiest person alive? All of this is perishable and fleeting. It will not bring true happiness. You must examine this question carefully. Is it for me or for the good of humanity? You only need what is necessary to fulfill your life's work. All else will be provided when needed, it will come of its own accord. The more possessions you have the more worries and concerns you have for keeping them and protecting them. Is this truly living? Worries cause mental agitation, agitation prevents peace of mind and without peace of mind there will be limited understanding of the teachings and limited ability to practice concentration and meditation. Worries and anxieties come from lack of understanding what is truly meaningful in life and ignorantly running after empty pleasures and distractions. Simplify your life! The goal of discovering the Self surpasses all worldly pleasures and all mental pleasures. Therefore, gradually make this the focus of your life and you will see how so many troubles fade and those adversities you would have led yourself into in the future are not gone forever.

"Consume pure foods and pure thoughts with pure hands, adore celestial beings, become associated with wise ones: sages, saints and prophets; make offerings to GOD."

—**From The Ancient Egyptian Stele of Djehuty-Nefer**

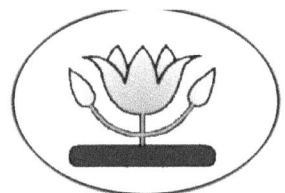

Question

How should an aspirant think about their personal practice, how much importance to assign to it and what should they do about taking the time to make the threefold observances when at work, and home, around others who follow other traditions, or when nobody knows what they are doing?

Setting Up The Personal Altar, To Practice The Daily Worship Program

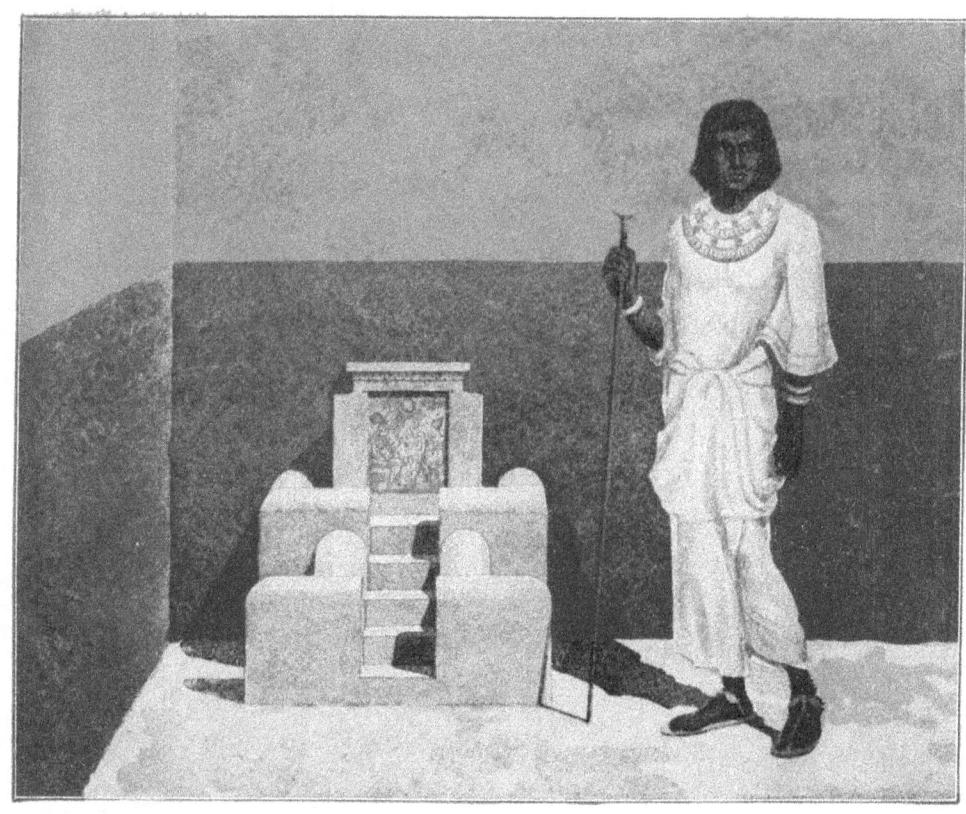

Above, image of an Ancient Egyptian man with a worship room and altar in his home (from 18th Dynasty)

Since ancient times it has been admonished to reserve a particular and exclusive part of the home (if possible an entire room) to setup an altar and practice the daily worship program. The Daily Worship Program consists of three worships during the day, one at dawn, one at noon and one at sunset. It may be practiced at times that are convenient but as close as possible to the prescribed optimal ritual times.

First, locate an area of your home where you can perform spiritual practices such as yoga exercises, prayers and meditations and not be disturbed. This area will be used only for yoga practice.

Now gather the basic materials needed to create your own altar. An altar is a place of worship which contains certain artifacts which hold specific spiritual symbolism that lead to spiritual awareness. The following items are to be considered as items for Neterian Worship and Spiritual practice. You are free to choose other items which resonate with your spiritual consciousness.

    1- Small **table**
    2- **Candle** - The candle holds deep mystical symbolism. It contains within itself all of the four elements of creation: fire, earth (wax in solid form), water (wax in liquefied form), and air. All are consumed in the burning process and all of them come together to produce light. This singular light represents the singular consciousness which shines throughout the entire universe. This light is the illumination which causes life to exist and it is the reason and source of the human mind. This light is life itself and life is God. Therefore, God is ever-present in the candle, in the universe (nature) and in your heart and mind.

Question

The Daily Worship Program consists of _____ worships during the day.

3- **Incense** - Incense invokes divine awareness through the sense of smell. When you perform spiritual practices and use a special incense consistently, every time that you smell the incense you will have divine thoughts and feelings even if you are not in the regular area of meditation. Therefore, select a fragrance which appeals to you and reflect within yourself that this is the fragrance of God in the same way as a flower emanates fragrance. Visualize that you are smelling divinity itself. From a personal perspective, also visualize that you are bathing in the fragrance in such a way that your scent will be attractive to the divinity you are propitiating.

4- **Ankh** - The Ankh is one of the most universal symbols expressing eternal life, the union of opposites and it was, and is used by the world religious traditions (ancient Egyptian religion, early Christianity, Indian religion and others. Visualize that this image carries with it the divine energy of life and existence such as what the gods and goddesses have who also carry it and that it will carry you through the struggles of life and on to survive into the higher planes of higher consciousness and Nehast, enlightenment.

5- **Sculpture or Iconic Image**, picture or other symbol of a Deity (as a symbol of the Supreme Being). This may be an ancient Egyptian Deity such as Heru, Aset, Asar, etc. Choose an icon according to your spiritual inclination. This will help you to develop devotion toward the Divine and will hasten your progress in yoga. This is called worship of God with name and form. This will be your tutelary divinity and your support as well as help in opening up the mysteries of other gods and goddesses and the mystery of the supreme and transcendental Divine Self. As you progress you will be instructed on how to worship the Divine in an abstract way without using any names or forms.

6- Two cups. One filled with water and the other empty to be used for pouring a libation.

7- A piece of material made of cotton or linen that is large enough to cover the altar when not in use.

8- Small **audio cassette recorder** (to lead your spiritual sessions). Or you may access the www.Egyptianyoga.com web site to play the worship program daily.

9- **Audio Recordings** of prayers, meditations, exercises, discourses from authentic Spiritual Preceptors.

10- **TIME TO PRACTICE THE MORNING WORSHIP** -For the first time initiation it is recommended that you reserve **one hour at four A.M.** and that you fast from 6 P.M the night before. This is also a good practice to continue during your regular morning worship and meditations.

11- Follow along with the daily worship program or if you do not have a recording read from the Devotional Worship Manual from the Morning Worship, or the Noon Worship or the Evening Worship.

12- To enhance the practice you can use a HETEP SLAB instead of the cups, for the libation part of the daily worship program. (see on next page)

Question

Choose an icon according to your spiritual _____.

In Ancient Egypt, the practice of sacrifice developed into an advanced performance of religious ritual in which live animals were not used. Instead, images were carved on stone or wooden ritual implements to represent the ideal of the cosmic force being propitiated. The Kemetic (Ancient Egyptian) philosophy holds that the image, *bes*, of an object is a higher reality relating to the ideal of the object. That is also the basis of the hieroglyphic texts which use iconographical symbols. Therefore, using the ideal form of the object elevates the sacrifice that much closer to perfection. A prime example of the sacrificial program is the use of the *hetep* offering table. The hetep offering table combines the libation offering with the food offering with mystical implications that relate to uniting the opposites of Creation in a similar way as the Shiva lingam-yoni of India.

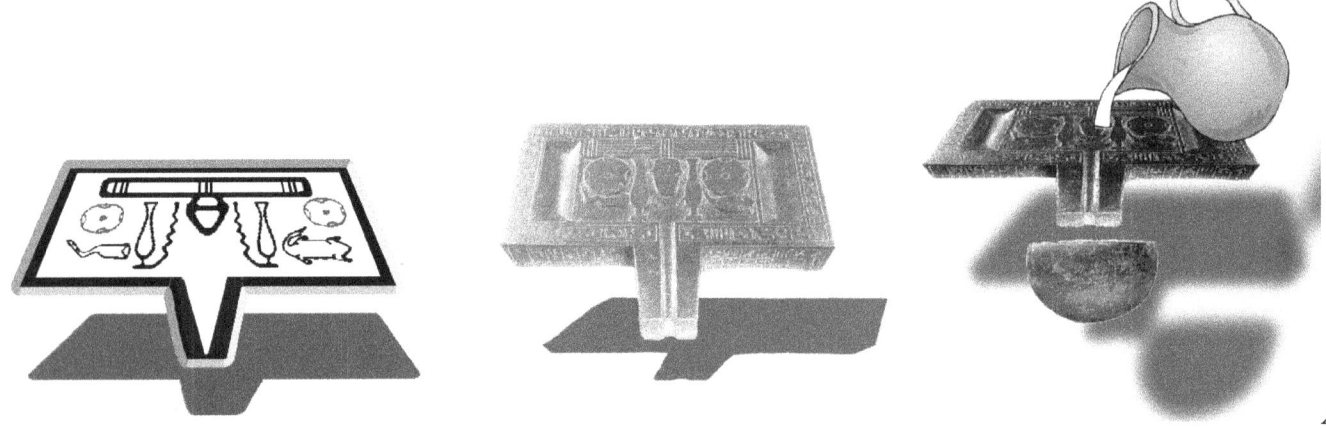

A

The "Hetep Slab" or Offering Table [above] is an important tantric symbol and ritual artifact from Ancient Egypt. It is typically composed of a stone slab with male ⌢, thigh, and female ⇔, duck, symbols carved into the top, along with the symbol of Supreme Peace, ⌴, or Hetep, which consists of a loaf of bread, ₒ, and an offering mat, ⌴, which was composed of woven reeds (in Pre-Dynastic times), and two libation vessels ⋂⋂. In ancient times the actual offering mat consisted of the articles themselves (loaf, thigh, duck and libation fluids (water, wine or milk) on a reed mat or wooden ritual offering table, but in Dynastic times (5,500B.C.E-400 A.C.E) the table top or slab contained the articles as engraved glyphs. The top of the table has grooves, which channel the libations around the offering toward the front and center of the table and then out through the outermost point of the protruding section. The hetep symbol, ⌴, means "rest", "peace" and "satisfaction" and when it is used in the hetep offering ritual it refers to the satisfaction of the neters (gods and goddesses) which comes from uniting the male and female principles into one Transcendental Being. The Hetep Offering Table can be seen in the innermost shrine of the Papyrus of Ani (Book of Coming Forth By Day of Ani) where the initiate Ani is shown making two offerings, one female and the other male. It can also be seen in the major museums around the world which have Ancient Egyptian collections. Below: A- operation of the offering table, B- Oldest known offering table from Ancient Egypt (c.4000 B.C.E.) Metropolitan museum-New York, C- Offering table from the papyrus of Ani. (Ancient Egypt c.1800 B.C.E.) D- Hetep offering of Auf Ankh (Ancient Egypt c.1800 B.C.E.)

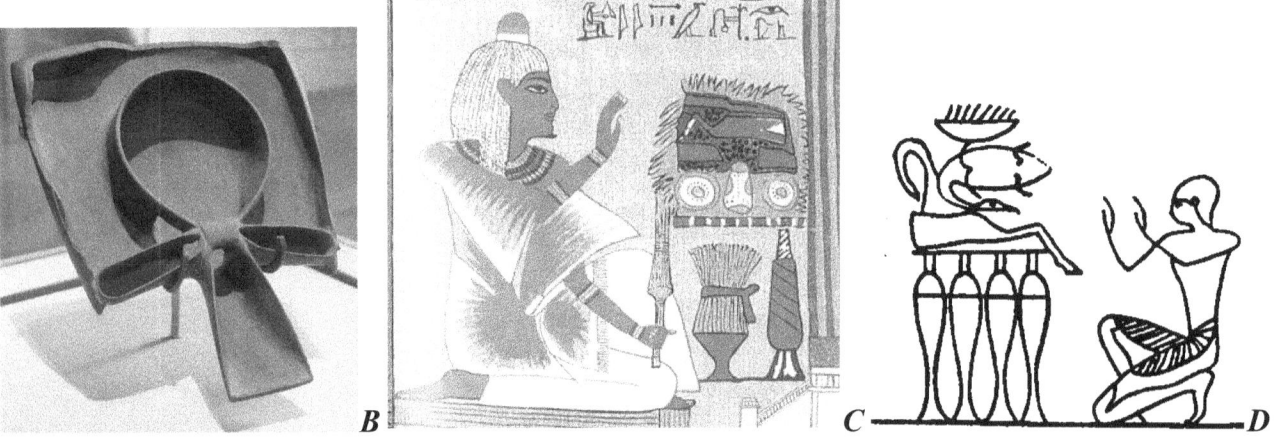

Question

Describe the "Hetep Slab"

Comportment and Demeanor As a Follower in the Spiritual Hall

In this essay, the topic will be how to conduct yourself as in initiate in the presence of the initiatic company, which is your Shedy group or in the presence of the spiritual preceptor. First of all, in ancient times when coming to a spiritual hall you would wash yourself before coming into the temple itself. This practice of the Ancient Egyptians is what later developed into the baptism ritual for the Christians. So you want to be cleansed, you must be cleansed physically, you must be cleansed in your mouth, in your speech, and you must cleansed in your mind. That means that you do not utter harsh words to anyone but if you utter harsh words to anyone you must resolve that issue before coming to the temple otherwise, your mind will be agitated and you will not draw the grace that the temple has to offer. You do not come in to the temple harboring thoughts of anger, hatred, greed, lust, jealousy, envy, and so forth. Therefore, you do not have sex before coming into the temple either. This is very disruptive to the experience of elevated spiritual vibrations. You do not eat meat before coming to the temple; it has its own worldly vibrations. You do not come to the temple with worldly possessions, you leave them at the door or put them over your coat or put them in your locker if you need one. You do not carry cell phones or pagers (beepers) you should not distract yourself or others. If you are the kind of person who does business 24 hours a day it simply means that you should be elsewhere doing that business.

Attending the class is very important to your spiritual instruction. You should attend any function prescribed by the teacher. The class is to be conducted in the manner that it has been prescribed and there should not be any deviations from that other than what has been allowed by the preceptor. It is set up that way, so that it would lead you in a proper way to develop your spiritual studies. Any deviations or adjustment are to be approved only by the preceptor and the reason for that is because you want to be managed in a proper way, you want to make sure that you are not going astray. It is the responsibility of the preceptor to shepherd you towards the correct practice and movement towards the Divine. What would happen if a train dwells? There are other students that study Egyptian Yoga Series in countries that do not have preceptorship at all, and it is great that they are making that effort. But it would be much better to also have authentic preceptorship. If this is done in a proper way it is guaranteed that you will succeed in your spiritual life.

Greeting the Spiritual Preceptor and The Term Seba

How do you greet and respect the Spiritual Preceptor. How should you approach a spiritual preceptor? When you come into the hall, when you are clean and with the right clothing, you've been allowed in to the courtyard of the temple. The first thing that you do is to prostrate yourself before the divine image and greet the priest or priestess. Prostration is being on your heels, but this time with your toes curled in, your hands in front of you resting on your elbows. Your forehead on the ground your face kissing the ground. Even if the Shrine is closed you will prostrate yourself in front of the Shrine and then take your seat. The Spiritual preceptor is known as 'Seba' in Kamitan spirituality. Sehu, another term, means spiritual counselor. Seba means preceptor, so that you can understand it, this term is similar to but not exactly the same as the Indian term 'guru'. The preceptor is greeted in the basic manner of this tradition, 'hotep' or 'hetep' whichever pronunciation you would like. The preferred manner of obeisance toward the spiritual preceptor is with both arms raised with hands facing outwards towards the preceptor and that is called the 'dua' posture. Dua means adoration and you have heard that word plenty of times in the chants: Dua Hetheru Netritaah, Dua Ra, Dua Ra Khepera, etc. And for greeting each other a simple hetep and a bow will do. This is the basic etiquette of the Shedy group.

For more insight into the term, Seba means star, it means an illuminating force, a shining object. Therefore the reason why preceptors are called Seba is because they illumine. Now, what do they illumine? They illumine the 'sebat' seba with the 't' at the end of it. In Kemetic literature, those of you who have began

NOTES:

You should try not to come in to the _____ harboring thoughts of anger, hatred, greed, lust, jealousy, envy, and so forth.

Write a brief essay on how to conduct oneself in the temple:

What is the meaning of the term Seba?

studying the writings, when you add a 't' to a word it makes if female. What all this means is that all of you as students are females, whether you are a male or female and the preceptor is male, whether the preceptor is male or female. What that means is that the illuminator is shining on you just like the sun shines on the moon, just as the moon, a symbol of mind, receives illumination from the sun, the student receives illumination from the teacher. That illumination is a reception or being in a female capacity just as in the sexes in an ordinary sexual relationship, the male is emitting and the female is receiving. The female receives and with that takes and creates a fertilized egg and brings forth life. In the same way the student is to allow their mind to become pregnant with the teachings and through the teachings eventually give birth to enlightened consciousness. That is the deep philosophy behind the term 'Seba'.

Similarly in India, the term 'guru' symbolizes illuminator, one who illumines the cave of heart or shines a light on there to see what is in there. In the Kemetic Culture and deep mysticism you have an artifact, which is called 'Seba-ur', Ur means great, therefore, it is 'the great illuminator.' The great illuminator is an instrument that you see being touched to the mouth in the opening of the mouth ceremony. This artifact is a symbol of a star constellation that used to be in the North Pole, there are many details about it. In short for now, for our purpose here and for your understanding, it means stars that do not move. If you were to see time-lapse photography of the north pole, you see that there are some stars that circulate around the north pole and go under the horizon and they come up again the next day. If you look at the North Pole, the North Pole does not go under the horizon, it stays above and further, it does not move. The North Pole does not change, just like the sun does not change, but the moon has phases. So when you are a student, you are changeable some days you have very good understanding of the teachings and you are with it and some days you are going along but your mind is locked up, or your emotions are getting the best of you, that means of you have lots of past impressions coming up, you have anger, hatred, greed, lust, jealousy, envy, etc., coming out of the unconscious mind that you need to deal with and cleanse. The teachings do not want you to feel angry or greedy and so forth. That is the mind changing and that is like the moon. When you continue to receive the teachings, receiving illumination one day you do not fluctuate anymore and is what the 'Seba-ur' means.

Sitting Postures

The next important point is your posture there are several postures that are allowed in the Kemetic culture. One is the cross-legged posture, the lotus posture or the half lotus posture, which are more difficult postures to do, granted. The other posture is sitting on a chair with your legs together and your hands on both sides of your tights that one is allowed also if you need to. Another one is sitting on the ground with your feet together as if you were sitting on a chair, with your feet together or the same posture and grasping your legs side to side and holding your legs together. These are all postures that you will see in the Kemetic culture. You do not extend your feet forward, especially toward the divinity or the Sage. You do not slough over or lay down. These kinds of postures will tend to lead you toward slumber and they will also tend to impair your reasoning capacity and your mental understanding. You have a Djed Pillar in your back and if that Djed Pillar is straight, that is, vertical with the ground it is like a tree, it goes straight up and so you too must be planted as a Djed Pillar. Another posture is sitting on your knees and your heels. These postures will all lead you to attentiveness, they will lead you to wakefulness, and these features are necessary when you attend a special lecture.

Any lecture by your spiritual preceptor is to be considered as "special" and deserves your undivided attention. Usually, you will not be expected to endure a posture for more than hour and also sometimes it is preferable not to have a back on your chair or to sit against a wall because you will be leaning and resting on the back (of the chair) and you do not want to be too comfortable because again you will falling asleep, so and so forth.

QUESTION

Name the different ways one can sit in the temple.

NOTES:

Respect for the Shrine and Conduct in the Temple

The shrine, is kept closed, expect during the time when the program is being conducted and actually the shrine is only open to initiates. The shrine will be there, but it will be closed only initiates are allowed to see the Divinity, only certain initiates are allowed to manipulate or handle the Divinity, the image of the Divinity. The reason for that is that people with impure hands, those people who are not pure as we said earlier, who have not purified the body, speech, and mind, carry worldly vibrations and they carry impressions of ignorance. The secrecy regarding the image of the Divinity is to develop awe and admiration from the masses and when initiates are finally allowed to see it they are consumed by its dazzling nature. By that time they have been schooled, and have been led to understand certain things about what they will see, certain things about the image, the headdress, the staff and other things that they are going to be seeing, ankhs, scepters, the colors, etc.

Going back to the relationship inside the Temple. You want to be silent rather than talkative, introverted rather than extroverted. You want to be dedicated, meditative, if you come to the Hall and the program has not started yet, you want to come in and sit down, prostrate, do whatever is necessary and take your seat quietly. You don't want to enter and be boisterous, rowdy or loud like 'hey, you see what I did the other day and this happen to me,' that is for people outside. Cacophony, yelling, loud mouth speech, etc. is for the outside world. You want to discover the inner world. This is not a social club or social party, this is not a place for you to come so you can have a membership card, so you can say you are an initiate and put on airs, looking down on others like 'I know these things, I am higher than you.'

You are not here so you can put on Kamitan jewelry, and clothing so that people can be looking at you and be watching you; that is egoism that is not initiation. You must be in a serious mind if you enter into initiation and I want to let know what it takes, for you to succeed. Coming to class once a week is great, that is more than 99% of what the world population does. You are already elevating yourself beyond the rest of the world, but in that top 1% how many people become enlightened? Maybe one thousandths of that one percent becomes enlightened. Are you going to be in the thousandths? This is what it takes, you want to read the books thoroughly and then you go back and read them again. There are lectures that are given on the texts, listen to those lectures again because if you listen to one lecture one time you are not going to get everything that is in it. You may have to listen to it three, four times or more. After a few months pass, you may want to go back and listen to it again. You will realize that something important that was said, you missed the first or second time around or now since you have evolved further, by the third listening, you are discovering a new nuance that applies to you in a whole new way. You should listen to the tapes until the teaching is inculpated deep in your mind and until you're conscious mind is cleansed, recall that three fold cleansing that we discussed earlier.

Again, a few other little points, the chanting, the divine singing etc. are very big parts of the Kemetic Culture as I have said before, it allows you to take the teaching, elevate it with your feeling and fly to meet the Divine with it. Devotion in your worship, Divine Love, is the essential key, but devotion without wisdom is, as I have said before, blind faith. Wisdom without devotion is dry intellectualism. After you learn to love this Divinity, if you do not know that Divinity, or how that Divinity relates to you, or what it is, how can you truly come close to the Divine? How can you love someone you do not even know? You must get to see a connection, develop a connection or feeling, and understand also. When feeling and understanding are harmonized and cultivated there is no stopping your spiritual evolution. You need to learn he chants by heart and this should not be too difficult if you are practicing them on a daily basis. In fact, it should become automatic, so you may use the sheets to begin with, but I want you to know that you have to put the sheets down, also eventually at least for the basic chants and prayers. Otherwise they will be like crutches, and that is not the ideal. If you do that it will not allow you to relax with it and to flow with it and this is something that needs to happen in your devotional feeling. The flow is going to constantly be interrupted and your mind will be constantly drawn into the paper and you need to be able to allow your thoughts as well as your feelings to flow towards the Divine in an unobstructed manner. The same goes for the drumming, cymbal playing or sistrum playing.

Question

How can you love someone you do not even _____?

Spiritual Clothing

The very clothing itself has spiritual meaning, the way the hair is done, and all of these different items carry a special mystical meaning. At the time of initiation, you should have been cleansed, and have your white or light colored clothing, upon entering the spiritual hall. You do not come to the spiritual hall with your lowly worldly clothing, you should have special clothes for the spiritual teachings. The garb is an absolute necessity, it is an augmentation, it is something that helps the practice. It is symbolic of putting on a new body, a new consciousness, a new birth, like the snake as it sheds its old skin and becomes reborn as it were into a new body and thereby has a new life in a bigger body. So too the aspirant has an expanded consciousness.

Part of the ritual of initiation is that you must be preparing yourself with the right clothing. It is taking a bath, it is making sure that you smell properly. In Kemetic philosophy, hygiene is of utmost importance for your health, not only physically but also for mental and physical health. If there is no hygiene there is going to distraction because you are going to have disease and disease will take you away from your spiritual disciplines. How are you going to come to a spiritual hall if you are on the bed, laid up with disease? In a practical sense it cannot work. Hygiene of your body, speech, and of your mind are the three main concerns for an initiate. What do you do when you go out in the street? You go out you do your business and take a shower when you come home. In the same way you should take a shower for your mouth, a shower for your mouth is uttering the Divine Chants, Divine Singing. The shower for your mind is the practice of meditation, it allows all that day activity to wash away, to be cleansed away.

Therefore just as you take a shower daily you should do your chants daily, you should do the meditation daily, and of course we have tapes that are already set up for that purpose, to help you to do your practices at home on a daily basis. You may be meeting once a week as a group, but on a daily basis as initiates you are expected to play the Morning Worship Tape and beyond that your are expected to enter into individual studies on the teachings, the philosophy. Taking your own initiative to follow up on teachings that you have received by the Spiritual Preceptor. This requires you to spend more time than just attending classes on Sunday and doing your morning worship. Like I have suggested previously, you can play lecture tapes on your way to work, in your car, or if you have a walk-man, a cassette player or any such devices.

Also, in your personal bodies you must realize that given the nature of the teachings that you are trying to learn that the body is not your ultimate abode. It is not your only existence. The perpetual worrying or running after the body, putting oils on the body and the body must have nice clothing to look good, then it must have jewelry, and it must have nice oils for the hair, special shampoo, and this and that, or tattoos, or piercing. All of this is counterproductive to the teaching and therefore, it is not enjoined in the teaching. This understanding excludes the spiritual clothing and certain other aspects. They have a spiritual symbolism that turn your mind actually towards the teaching, but not including piercing, not including use of chemicals on the body that transform the way your body naturally wants to manifest itself. Things that have a healthful nature are allowed. Things like synthetic chemicals for bleaching the skin, dying the hair, or straightening the hair; or things that will be make you unnaturally sexually alluring are all counterproductive to the teachings.

Question

Hygiene of your _____, _____, and of your _____ are the three main concerns for an initiate.

How to Overcome Failure on the Spiritual Path

Question: Having heard the teaching and after some time if you have not having attained spiritual enlightenment what is there to do?

Many aspirants study the teaching for some time, even years, and find that they have not achieved the ultimate goal of which the teachings speak, that great *Nehast,* the spiritual awakening that bestows the knowledge of nature and the Divine, that wisdom that opens the doors to eternity, that teaching that bestows immortality, supreme joy, peace and God consciousness which is spoken about so much and is the objective of all spiritual aspirants worldwide. What should an aspirant do if she or he finds her/him self in this predicament? The aspirant should take recourse to

1. Repeated effort and
2. Dispassion (becoming free from delusion about the world and desire and hatred) which clouds the intellect.
3. devotion with form
    a. this secures divine grace-

<u>Repeated effort means:</u> at this level of practice (in the teaching for some time-even years), not just listening to the teachings and going about one's worldly business. It means diligence in the practice of the teachings and the disciplines enjoined by the teachings. There must be uncompromising meticulousness and fastidiousness and strictness in the practice. Not sporadic or irregular practice. Some aspirants practice salad-bar spirituality, picking and choosing what they want to do. Some come to some lectures, some rituals, some meditation gatherings, some meetings and then wonder why they have not succeeded, yet they have not attended to the teaching in a full way. There will be only limited success until the teaching and its disciplines are attended to fully by an aspirant. Some aspirants allow gaps of years in the practice of the teachings, falling in and out of worldly entanglements. This is not the path to the ultimate success because it is not the highest and best practice of the teachings- *Sdjm* –heeding the teaching. Even while living in the world an aspirant must find a way to handle the worldly responsibilities –this is righteous and proper-for without this there is no basis for practice of the teachings. But worldly responsibilities are not to be pursued beyond necessity.

"Neither let prosperity put out the eyes of circumspection, nor abundance cut off the hands of frugality; they that too much indulge in the superfluities of life, shall live to lament the want of its necessaries."
-Ancient Proverb of Shetaut Neter

Worldly responsibilities that are performed for the sake of promoting spiritual practice are to be considered Divine actions, -part of the spiritual disciplines as opposed to those that are performed for the sake of promoting more pursuit of worldly pleasures and worldly desires. Repeated effort also means working to become less entangled with the world and to lead a simple life-pay off mortgages, get a car for transportation and not as a status symbol, seeking the company of spiritually minded (others who study the teaching-not religious people) people as opposed to worldly minded, living within one's means, etc. Having taken care of the worldly duties-providing for ones food, shelter and health- the attention is to be turned towards the teaching exclusively, meaning that the actions are to be performed for the sake of the Divine and not for the egoistic self.

NOTES:

Sdjm means _____ the teaching.

After practicing for many years and not becoming enlightened the recourse an aspirant should take is: _____

Lack of Dispassion- without dispassion the teaching will not the mind and second step of assimilation of the teaching will not occur or will occur imperfectly and the third stage will not be possible at all. There are three stages in the process of study of the teaching, Listening, Reflection and Meditation. Reflection is the second stage. When the teaching has been heard then it needs to be reflected upon deeply and this reflection process leads to assimilation of the teaching into the depth of the mind and finally there is meditation on the teaching, the single-minded and singular experience of the deeper meaning of the teaching in one's own experience.

Maturity to Succeed in the teaching does not occur until there is sufficient frustration with the pursuit of worldly desires. A person's capacity to practice dispassion emerges when they realize the futility of trying to fulfill their egoistic desires through worldly pleasures and so dispassion is a reaction to frustration but if the dispassion is based on ignorance-the lack of spiritual teaching, then it will be short-lived. That person will experience dispassion only for a short time and then be back to worldly pursuits.

"Neither let prosperity put out the eyes of circumspection, nor abundance cut off the hands of frugality; they

that too much indulge in the superfluities of life, shall live to lament the want of its necessaries."

-Ancient Proverb of Shetaut Neter

Dispassion is the gradual freedom achieved when the mind becomes released from the mood swings caused by desire and hatred due to ignorance about the world and passionate desire to fulfill desires through the world of time and space. These desires are a product of a deluded mind that does not realize the futility of trying to fulfill desires through a fleeting world of human experiences. This search causes the mind to be clouded with ignorance and there can be no peace due to the constant mental swings themselves and the deluded concepts that the mind subscribes to. The movements of the mind cloud the intellect and prevent right thinking. The ignorant concepts act as impenetrable canvases or images of the world in accordance with the desires of the mind. This renders the world not as it is but as a deluded notion of reality based on the internal egoistic notions and desires. In this state of mind objects and worldly pursuits are chased after without regard for truth because the desire has blotted out the negative aspects and painted a picture of happiness in the object or pursuit. This deluded notion renders the mind incapable of assimilating the teachings in a proper way.

"God sheds light on they who shake the clouds of Error from their soul, and sight the brilliancy of Truth, mingling themselves with the All-sense of the Divine Intelligence, through love of which they win their freedom from that part over which Death rules, and has the seed of the assurance of future Deathlessness implanted in him. This, then, is how the good will differ from the bad."
-Ancient Proverb of Shetaut Neter

NOTES:

When does maturity to succeed in the teachings occur?

Divine Grace = God does not grant Nehast (Spiritual awakening-enlightenment) This is not within God's power to give. As a spark of the Divine every human being is essentially one with God and as such partakes in Divine Power. The soul, as that spark, has led itself to ignorance and so by itself must lead itself to awakening. Practicing devotion to God has the effect of turning the mind towards the Divine and this leads to purity of feeling and thinking. Essentially it is a worship of the Divinity within oneself. When the divinity within is worshipped as opposed to the world, it allows that divinity to emerge as the preeminent aspect of life and the mind AWAKENS to its presence and the true nature of the personality which is not the egoistic notion but the heretofore unknown Divine Spirit-God within. Devotional exercises bestow propitious conditions to practice and advance in spiritual attainment. God does not grant enlightenment but only opens the door. Propitious conditions includes peace of mind, encounters with spiritual preceptors, reduction of pressure of egoistic tendencies that act as obstacles to spiritual attainments. When Divine Grace dawns the aspirant gains spiritual strength and increasing desire to study and practice the teaching as well as increasing pleasure and fulfillment through the practice and increasing dispassion about the worldly objects and worldly desires. Divine Grace is propitiated through Devotion to the Divine and Right Action-righteousness.

"Seekest thou God, thou seekest for the Beautiful. One is the Path that leadeth unto It - Devotion joined with Knowledge."

-Ancient Proverb of Shetaut Neter

Devotion to God allows the depth of the teaching to be revealed. Approaching the teaching intellectually will only promote a superficial understanding and therefore a limited attainment. Intellectual study allows the teaching to be thought about but this thinking process can become circular if the depth of the teaching is not approached. Devotion-Divine Love towards God allows the depth of the teaching to be approached. In essence the teaching must be felt as well as known. Intellectual knowledge must be augmented by feeling the teaching. The feeling aspect of the soul, when tapped into, does not allow the intellectual aspect to become deluded. In fact, it will plague the intellect with insecurities, torment the intellect with doubts until the right path is pursued this is the deeper conscience of a person-whose source is their own soul. This cannot occur of the divine feeling is dulled due to delusion and worldly desire. Devotional exercises and rituals allow the intellectual teaching to be experience as well as thought.

"O behold with thine eye God's plans. Devote thyself to adore God's name. It is God who giveth Souls to

millions of forms, and God magnifyeth whosoever magnifieth God."

-Ancient Proverb of Shetaut Neter

Super-conscious state – in order for the process of spiritual evolution to occur there must be experience of the superconscious state of mind. The mind must experience going beyond the bounds of its own constrictive concepts and desires and the world of time and space. Otherwise, the teaching and the feeling of the spiritual process will remain short of the highest attainment no matter how pious the person may be or how elevated the mind and personality may appear to be. All the disciplines lead to a meditative experience in which time and space are transcended and all-encompassing, eternal existence and unlimited expanded consciousness is discovered. First in small measure and eventually in full splendor. Even a short glimpse which is merely a preview, unlocks lifetimes of mental fetterings and sparks the true awakening if the final phase of the march towards spiritual awakening.

Question

Divine Love towards God allows the depth of the teaching to be _____.

Meditation is the key to opening the mind to the experience of superconsciousness and this can only be achieved when the mind and personality has been cleansed of delusion, passion, attachment for worldly objects and desires. This purity leads to spiritual strength and spiritual strength is the key factor needed to attain entry into the superconscious state. In order to attain the highest meditative state, concentration and extended practice of mental focus is required. Without mental purity, and peace concentration is impossible and the superconscious state will elude even the cleverest intellect.

Spiritual Strength – In order to succeed on the spiritual path an aspirant needs spiritual strength. Spiritual strength is the strength that emerges when the mind is freed of ignorance, delusion and passion. The ignorant, deluded and passionate mind is fettered by its conscious and subtle desires and misconceptions. The conscious desires lead to worldly pursuits but this process, being unfulfilled, leaves residues of unfulfilled desire and also produces new subtle desires for other pursuits (if this desire did not work, maybe another will-etc. For Example: the deluded mind may reason thus- If a blue car did not make me happy, maybe a red one will) and these all become lodged in the unconscious level of mind. This constitutes a continued fettering of the mind in the present and in the future. These fetter the minds power because each subtle desire locks a portion of will power with itself in the unconscious level of mind. So even a person who appears to be free of desires may harbor these in the unconscious mind and thereby be weak willed. Such a person cannot resist worldly desires, nor can they sit still for meditation because thoughts constantly emerge to disturb the mind and even if thought do not seem to be emerging at some particular time there are energy disturbances throughout the body and there is illusory discomfort and the person claims they cannot succeed in meditation. So mental restlessness due to subtle desires, or energies must be resolved (cleansed and transcended by the mind) in order to succeed on the spiritual path. This is done by

    a-practice of devotion to god

    b- practice of right action

    c- practice of dispassion and detachment for the world

    d- practice of attachment to the teaching

    e- repeated effort in the above (a-d) until there is ultimate success

Desires are of three types: Heavenly (Maatian), Worldly (Un-Maatian) and mixed. Those who seek success on the spiritual path must turn away from the worldly to the mixed and then from the mixed to the Divine. When Maatian (principles of right action based on truth) actions are practiced the personality becomes purified, the mind becomes unburdened from vises and egoistic tendencies. Then the personality is capable of understanding and experiencing the higher consciousness talked about in the teachings. Therefore, the desire for worldly attainments should be replaced with desire for spiritual attainments in the form of increasing Divine Love, increasing dispassion and increasing peace and desire to study the teachings and be in the company of those who espouse it. Thus, spiritual evolution entails turning away from worldly desire and towards desire to attain spiritual awakening. Therefore, desire is not the problem, what is the problem is what is desired. The right desire leads to freedom and enlightenment. The wrong desire leads to ignorance, delusion, fettered bondage to the world and its accompanying virtually boundless source of human suffering, unfulfillment and sorrow.

Question

The desire for worldly attainments should be replaced with desire for _____ attainments.

<u>Diligence on the Path-</u> Mature aspirants need to grow up- arrange their priorities, conserve resources and invest in their own evolution, pay their dues (seminar fees, etc.), not leaving each other and the temple to shoulder the burdens, drop childish worldly entanglements that distract from the teaching, drop competing philosophies and infantile teachings that foment confusion so they can concentrate on what they proclaim to be following. Diligence on the spiritual path is not independent self-will. Those who want to practice salad bar spirituality or seek the advice of oracles or create their own independent classes should do so on their own. One cannot be a Shemsu in this way, by mixing teachings, following confused ideologies, following popular culture as the individual finding his or her own way. These are illusions of a decadent time that were always there but now in epidemic proportions due to the modern capacity to have a plethora of sensory bombardments, misinformations and complexities which play on the ignorant and distracted mind. Aspirants have no choice as to what the practice of the teaching needs to be in order to attain success. They do have a choice in the intensity of their level of practice and devotion to the teaching and these determine to the level or degree of success that is attained and when.

If you want to succeed be consistent with your studies. Do not attend classes sometimes, practice the postures sometimes, meditate sometimes, and then also carry on in the world as a worldly person. Do you eat sometimes, sleep sometimes? As these things are done daily so should the teaching be done as well. If you want success concentrate on this teaching and drop others. Follow the instructions carefully and meticulously and when there is faltering, pick yourself up and try again and again. Practice the teachings in this manner until the goal is attained, no matter how long it takes or where you need to go to receive it.

<u>A qualified aspirant</u> will not wait for the teaching but will make a way for it. He or she will not sit around hoping to find a teacher. The first task is to make yourself a qualified aspirant, purify yourself physically and mentally and be diligent in the studies under the guidance of your own conscience in the beginning, But there is a time when you must seek out a teacher. You must have the attitude that if I must travel to the other side of the world then that is what needs to be done. If you do not want to leave your family, your friends, job, etc. to pursue the teaching and enlightenment then you should not because you will not succeed even if you forced yourself, so realize that you are not yet fit for advancement in the teachings. Even college students leave home to pursue their dreams. What could be said about those who do not want to pursue the greatest goal of life because they are holding on to worldly things?

These are the keys for all who wish to excel in the teaching but they should be the special focus for all who have studied the teaching for some time and yet find themselves without success beyond a specific point. A DETERMINED ASPIRANT MUST SEE THE ENDEAVOR OF SPIRITUAL AWAKENING TO ITS END. If this is not done the aspirant will forever wander in the wilderness of life, deluded and suffering or self-aggrandized, believing they have attained when in reality they are projecting on the world their notion of reality reflecting within their illusion of sagehood. Such personalities walk the earth without the necessary humility to realize their own degraded state and thereby deprive themselves of the illuminating association with an authentic teacher. Others, convinced they have practiced correctly do not seek out counseling and so their dispassion turns to morose and sometimes even morbid discontent with all things including the teaching.

Question

Those who want to practice salad bar _____ or seek the advice of oracles or create their own independent classes should do so on their own.

How should an aspirant think about their spiritual path when they encounter failure to meet the instructions of the teaching or they fail to execute their own desired level of practice?

The Spiritual Checklist

In the last issue I began a two part series on how to overcome failure on the spiritual path. This brought up certain issues that are very important for aspirants to understand. Many times as aspirants get into the teaching for some time they may get into a rut as it were. They practice as many of the teachings and disciplines as they can but as they do that sometimes they get to a point where they must drop certain disciplines in order to practice others due to lack of time. In this circumstance a certain irregularity in the practice of the disciplines develops and the quality of all the disciplines suffers. The worldly activities and relations become intermingled with the disciplines and the spiritual program becomes haphazard. The aspirant may believe they are doing so many disciplines, chanting, classes, exercises, diet, etc. but in reality they may come for class once a week, do postures once or twice a week, take vitamins three times a week, do morning worship twice a week, etc. then next week these disciplines are left our in favor of others. What results is a situation where so many things are being done but the quality of those things is degraded and they do not have the effect of purifying the mind and shielding it from worldly entanglements. In fact the disciplines when practiced in this way can have the opposite effect and lead to a degraded personality because the effort put into the practice and then frustration when the feelings of anger, hatred, greed, lust, etc. still remain leads to the idea that the teaching does not work or the aspirant may simply get caught in the worldly experiences. Then the aspirant will come back to the teacher and ask what they can do, where did they go wrong, etc. They receive encouragement and advice but then the cycle begins all over again and there is no ultimate progress. This is because at that stage what is most important is to practice the disciplines. Spiritual counseling is necessary sometimes but if the disciplines are not practiced the counseling will also not be effective. For this reason the following list has been prepared. It contains the practices and disciplines that should be taken care of so that aspirants may understand when they are actually practicing the teaching and when they are actually not. Before calling the preceptor look at this list and see if you are truly following the instructions or not. If you find that you are not then make the necessary adjustment in your spiritual practice. Then if assistance is still needed call for advice. Keep a spiritual diary/journal along with the table below. Note over time how your personality is changing and seek to avoid the mistakes of the past. See the book Initiation into Egyptian Yoga for more details. HTP

In the table below you must be able to check off ✓each item daily, weekly, monthly and annually in order to consider yourself as practicing the teaching of Shetaut Neter and Sema Tawi. It is important to practice the daily disciplines daily because this regular practice will be most effective to transform the mind. However, if one practice is missed then double up (to make up) the next day if possible or on the weekend, etc. do not say, "the yesterday is passed and I cannot go back so let me forget about it and start today."

NOTES:

How should an aspirant think about their spiritual checklist and how diligent should they try to be with it?

An aspirant should keep a _____ diary.

Essential Daily practices		Essential Weekly practices		Essential Monthly practices		Essential Annual practices	
	✓		✓		✓		✓
Nutrition: vitamins and supplements		Keep company with elevated personalities at least 1 hour per week		Give 1/10 donation		Attend annual conference	
Nutrition: vegetarian diet		Selfless service 1 hour					
No smoking		Fasting 1 day per week		Celibacy: no sex more than once per month**		Make annual observance of the Kemetic New Year	
No drugs or alcohol							
Daily worship							
8 hours sleep							
Go to bed by 12 am							
Wake up early by 8 am							
Study of spiritual scripture- Ex. reading systematically the *Pert M Hru* text							
Abstain from company with negative personalities							
Silent meditation 20 minutes twice daily							
Practice breathing rhythmically 10 minutes twice daily							
Practice physical exercises 15 minutes daily							
*Observe the 42 Precepts of Maat (especially no lying, cheating, stealing, killing, hurting others***, etc.							
No talking for 1 hour (during waking hours)							

*At the end of the day read 42 Precepts of Maat and see if any were broken practice penitence for each transgression on an equal time basis (if the transgression lasted 1 hour practice the penitence to redress that transgression for at least 1 hour). First make a vow and then practice a penance for a period of time- you must observe the full period of the vow of penitence. Example of penitence: 1 hour of silence, not watching television for one day, not going to beach for one week, not eating the ice cream, not playing the music, not meeting with friends, etc. (Choose one penitence per transgression, it must be something that your ego desires otherwise it will have no effect on your personality. The idea is to assert your will over your ego by subjecting it to the regulation of Maat and not the unconscious desires. See your penitence as an austerity, a sacrifice period to redress the transgression and purify the heart.

**If this practice has not been kept skip you planned encounter of the future. Sleep separate from your partner for a period of time. Keep in mind that for advanced practice celibacy is to be observed for a 7 year period. Monastic aspirants maintain separate sleeping quarters. The advice given above is for householder aspirants. Remember that children will add more responsibilities and duties to your life that will leave less time for the practice of the teachings so use appropriate contraception in accordance with your desired level of practice. See book *Egyptian Tantric Yoga*.

***If you hurt someone by word or deed apologize to them and practice the austerity in * above. If you hurt someone by thought simply recognize the error and practice the austerity

NOTES:

THE TRADITION OF INITIATION

Those who are seriously interested in pursuing spiritual life should follow the instructions given in the previous section, seeking to purify themselves so as to become proper vessels to recognize and understand the teacher when he or she arrives. There is a tendency sometimes to engage in the flights of emotionality and in the psychic contacts that can be made when you begin to discover the inner dimensions of the mind. Sometimes aspirants believe they have encountered genuine divine personalities not realizing that these are expressions of their own mental creations as in a dream. Others believe that since they have experienced certain psychic "energies" or have developed certain psychic abilities, that this in and of itself constitutes spiritual enlightenment.

You must clearly understand that psychic phenomena do not necessarily signify or accompany spiritual enlightenment such as we are discussing here. Spiritual enlightenment is nothing short of mystical union with God. Therefore, while people may exhibit great feats of psychic nature or amazing control of bodily functions such as living without food for weeks or months or holding the breath for hours, etc., these are not to be automatically equated with spirituality and indeed may not have anything to do with spirituality in regard to the particular person who possesses such powers. Nevertheless, a spiritually enlightened personality may possess some such powers or may not. In any case, only one who is a genuinely advanced or an advancing spiritual personality can discern the difference. Thus, you must strive to purify yourself and dispel the illusions and misconceptions in your mind as to what constitutes true spirituality so that you may be led to the true spiritual teacher. Seek out those who exhibit compassion, patience, dispassion, equanimity of mind and selflessness. These are advanced psychic powers although they are not normally considered in this way. A stark contrast can be seen between ordinary egoistic human beings who think of providing for themselves and the pleasures of the body at the expense of others (the ignorant and worldly minded), and the more spiritually advanced individuals. The qualities of the ignorant, discontent, desire, hard-heartedness, distraction, mental agitation, restlessness, selfishness, etc., lead to experiences of pain, disappointment and frustration in life whereas the qualities of a spiritually advancing personality, selflessness, contentment, peacefulness, detachment from worldly possessions and relationships, etc., lead to greater levels of inner peace and self-discovery. These allow the mind to sink to deeper and deeper levels revealing the true nature of one's own being.

In the spiritual realm, you may encounter the divine in the form of God, Goddess, or an archetypal divine being. You may also experience this realm as wholeness, light, freedom, an awakening, etc. You need to understand that as you tread the path of initiatic science, you will need to gradually let go of all your mental concepts and notions of spirituality. This means that whatever you discover is to be understood as a relative reality because it is being perceived through the mind and senses which are limited.

If you do not have a specific spiritual preceptor who is versed in the spiritual disciplines of Yoga, the most important idea you need to keep in mind is your conviction to attain the highest. You must honestly and ardently ask for assistance and guidance while offering all of your activities and feelings to the Divine. As you learn about the various yogic paths, you will begin to develop a feeling for which course suits your personality. This is the reason why there are so many paths of yoga (devotional, wisdom, action, life force development, etc.). The process of becoming established on your personal path may involve a lot of ups and downs, trial and error, however you must be assured that if you follow through you will eventually reach the goal you have set.

Thus, self-initiation involves your decision to make the mystic path of yoga your life's endeavor. You must develop a strong desire to discover who you are and what the world is and you must have a deep rooted conviction that it is possible for you to understand and apply the principles and disciplines of yoga to your life, regardless of your life situation. At some point you may want to become formally initiated by a particular spiritual preceptor. This means that you have decided to come into closer association with the teaching as espoused by that teacher and that you are desirous of aligning yourself with the spiritual tradition of that teacher.

There are teachers who specialize in certain aspects of yoga disciplines. For example, a spiritual preceptor may focus on yoga through the wisdom teachings. This implies, studying, reflecting and rationalizing in order to develop a

Question

whatever you discover is to be understood as a relative reality because it is being perceived through the mind and senses which are _____.

subtle intellect which will be able to discover the spiritual truth. Another spiritual preceptor may focus on developing and disciplining the physical body through physical exercises and breathing exercises in order to achieve the same goal. Another may focus on prayer, and another on meditation, etc. However, if you find a preceptor who is well versed in Integral Yoga, which is the combination of these main yogic paths, you should not need to search further for other teachers.

In the meantime, apply yourself to the teachings to the best of your understanding and if possible, associate with others who are honest seekers on the path of self-discovery. Finding those around you who are sincerely interested in practicing yoga for spiritual development can be a powerful means to spiritual growth. When people come together, their energies are multiplied toward the task which they have chosen to undertake. This is also true of spiritual practice. Therefore, those who meet and help each other can keep the enthusiasm and level of interest up in positive as well as hard times. Also, in a group setting, the subtle vibrations are more strongly attuned to the study process which in turn helps the process of concentration and understanding. The group learning process is a powerful practice which helps toward the goal of purification of the heart, especially when it is conducted under the guidance of a spiritual preceptor.

The Ritual of Initiation

Rituals are a powerful process which can lead the mind toward spiritual thoughts and aspirations or toward pain and sorrow in life. People cling to ignorance by constantly seeking for pleasure and fulfillment in the world of time and space through human relationships, wealth, possessions, etc. Examples of negative rituals are: going to the video store, watching television, gossiping, partying or going to the movie theater in search of excitement. In the course of ordinary life you may experience these but if you rely on them as a source of pleasure and happiness you are bound for disappointments. All of life's activities are ritualistic to some degree. Every day we repeat many actions such as eating, sleeping, going to work, school or watching television. Other activities are less frequent but just as ritualistic; these include marriage, childbearing, etc. The basis of society's rituals is custom and habit. Society teaches and socializes young individuals into the activities it deems acceptable and thereby societal rituals develop. Rituals can be bad or good according to the level of spiritual realization within the individual as well as the society as a whole. If a society allows exploitation of some of its members, then rituals and customs develop which affirm that belief system. When society developed the materialistic view of life and discounted the spiritual values, material values became part of the general culture. Thus, pursuing material wealth and the experience of sensual pleasures have become the most commonly practiced rituals in modern day society. This is reflected in business, government and in the family way of life at all levels of society. These rituals are all performed toward perishable goals and thus can never satisfy the inner need of the soul. This movement constitutes a movement in ignorance which leads to further ignorance. While religious rituals are also in the realm of human activity, if performed with growing levels of understanding and devotion toward the Divine, they will lead to greater and greater peace and self-knowledge. Therefore, the Sages and Saints have enjoined several rituals, prayers and words of power to help spiritual aspirants turn the mind toward spiritual realization rather than toward perishable worldly attainments which will inevitably lead to disappointments, pain and sorrow.

Question

All of life's activities are _____ to some degree.

Initiation With a Spiritual Preceptor

In essence the entire program of study in Yoga is an initiatic ritual. However, a specific ritual of initiation is additionally efficacious since it serves to establish a subtle connection between teacher and disciple which fosters greater understanding through personal contact. It allows the aspirant to develop a devotional feeling toward the teacher and the teachings which relate to the *Self*. It engenders a mystic force towards spiritual aspiration even when done alone. Essentially, initiation is an expression of a person's personal conviction and desire to engage in a lifestyle which will lead to spiritual transformation. It is a commitment to a process of learning spiritual teaching and its practice. The initiation ritual performed with a Spiritual Preceptor also fosters a mystic link between an aspirant and his or her hekau and everything else related to the spiritual practice because it causes a deeper mental impression of their divine nature. This is especially important in the practice of chanting or hekau repetition. The hekau acts to cleanse the heart (mind) and it sets up positive vibrations which calm the mind and awaken spiritual feeling. Chanting elevates the mind and lifts it to transcendental levels.

The initiation ritual is usually accompanied by certain ceremonial rites and specific instruction on how chanting works and the procedure for uttering words of power. A specific hekau is given to an initiate based on the individual's spiritual inclination, attitudes and level of evolution. Initiations may be performed for individuals or for groups. A spiritual aspirant will be drawn to a Spiritual Preceptor on the basis of internal spiritual sensitivity. At some point in life a person will look for someone who can understand him or her and lead them on the spiritual path.

In ancient times those desiring to learn from a spiritual teacher would come to them with humility and reverence. They would bring fruits or firewood to help sustain the teacher and his or her efforts in disseminating the teaching. In Ancient Egypt the people and the government would support the Temples so that the spiritual upliftment of the country might be insured. Therefore, when you approach a teacher bring an offering. This may be a symbolic object but realizing that it represents your inner desire to grow spiritually and respect for the teachings you will receive. Also, come with patience and a spirit of joy. Then you will discover the true meaning of what the teachings really mean. This does not happen overnight. Fanaticism is not a part of real spiritual evolution. It is a hindrance. True spiritual evolution occurs in degrees. There is a Yoga parable given to illustrate this point. An aspirant went to a spiritual preceptor and asked for initiation into the teachings. The preceptor said "Alright, come to the temple and study the scriptures, attend my lectures and practice what I tell you." The aspirant said "Oh no, I don't have time for that. I want liberation from this miserable world now. Why will you withhold the teachings from me?" The preceptor replied "Very well, I will give you initiation into the teachings this evening. I will come to your house this evening but you must prepare the special food offering to your preceptor." That evening, the preceptor came and was greeted by the aspirant. The aspirant had set everything up and offered the preceptor a seat. The aspirant brought the food offering to the preceptor and the preceptor took out a bowl for the aspirant to put the food into. The aspirant was about to place the food in the bowl when he noticed that it was full of muck and insects so he said: "Please oh venerable sir, let me wash your bowl and then I will place the food into it." The preceptor replied: "No, that's alright, I will eat from this bowl the way it is." The aspirant was astonished and replied: "How can you expect me to put your food into that dirty bowl, I cannot do that." The preceptor replied: "How can you expect me to teach you the highest spiritual wisdom if you will not cleanse the vessel of your mind?" Immediately the aspirant understood the teaching and fell at the feet of the preceptor and pledged to follow his instruction from then on. The aspirant should realize that any endeavor in life requires instruction. Many fall under the delusion that the spiritual path can be accomplished without the help of a spiritual preceptor. All means should be used to learn but there is no better way than attending classes and receiving instruction from an authentic spiritual teacher. Then only through humility and total devotion is it possible to truly advance.

QUESTION

When you approach a teacher bring an _____.

NOTES:

What are You Being Initiated Into?

Those who wish to become *Shemsu Neter* (followers of the Kamitan (Ancient Egyptian) spiritual teaching, are initiated into *Shetaut Neter* and *Smai Tawi*. Shetaut Neter is the religion and its mythic teachings based on the varied traditions centered around the different gods and goddesses. Smai Tawi are the yogic disciplines, techniques or technologies used to transform a human being. These disciplines promote a transformation through a movement that purifies the personality and renders it subtle enough to perceive the transcendental spiritual reality beyond time and space. This is a movement from ignorance to enlightenment, from mortality and weakness to immortality and supreme power, to discover the Absolute from whence the gods and goddesses and all Creation arose. This is a movement towards becoming one with the universe and the consciousness behind it which is eternal and infinite. This is the lofty goal of initiation. So those who tread this path must be mature and virtuous as well as strong, physically, mentally and emotionally. The purpose of the religion and disciplines is to promote purity of heart and virtue and these lead to higher realization and spiritual enlightenment. Therefore, the next section will present an overview of Shetaut Neter and how it relates to Smai Tawi. The following section will present an overview of the Smai Tawi disciplines. For details on these areas see the books:

For Shetaut Neter see the book *The Book of Shetaut Neter* by Muata Ashby

For Smai Tawi see the books related to the particular discipline

>Wisdom Discipline: *The Mysteries of Aset (Isis)* by Muata Ashby
>Meditation Discipline: *Meditation The Ancient Egyptian Path to Enlightenment* by Muata Ashby
>Action Discipline: *The Wisdom of Maati* by Muata Ashby
>Feeling Discipline: *The Path of Divine Love* by Muata Ashby
>Life Force Discipline: *The Serpent Power* by Muata Ashby

NOTES:

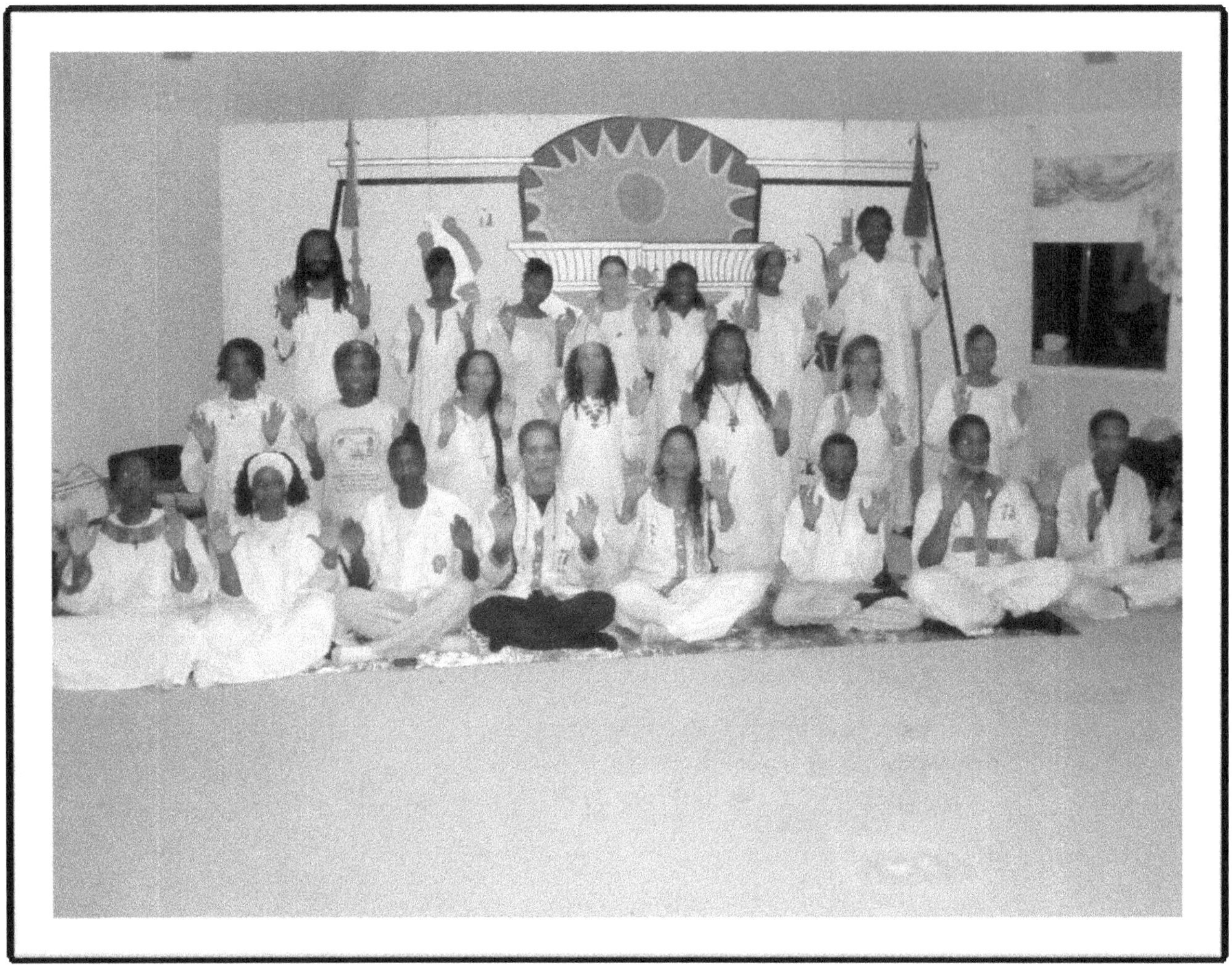

HTP
(Peace)

www.ingramcontent.com/pod-product-compliance
Lightning Source LLC
Chambersburg PA
CBHW081130170426
43197CB00017B/2814